Leslie&Susannah
Kenton

Authentic
Woman

A GUIDE TO BEAUTY, BODY&BLISS

Leslie&Susannah Kenton

Authentic Woman

A GUIDE TO BEAUTY, BODY&BLISS

Photography by Leslie Kenton

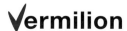

First published in Great Britain in 2005

1 3 5 7 9 10 8 6 4 2

First published by Vermilion, an imprint of Ebury Press

Random House UK Ltd, Random House, Vauxhall Bridge Road, London SW1V 2SA

Random House Australia (Pty) Limited, 20 Alfred Street, Milsons Point, Sydney, New South Wales 2061, Australia

Random House New Zealand Limited, 18 Poland Road, Glenfield, Auckland 10, New Zealand

Random House (Pty) Limited, Endulini, 5a Jubilee Road, Parktown 2193, South Africa

Random House UK Limited Reg. No. 954009 www.randomhouse.co.uk

A CIP catalogue record for this book is available from the British Library

Editor: Yvette Brown Design: Two Associates

ISBN: 0091898668

Papers used by Vermilion are natural, recyclable products made from wood grown in sustainable forests.

Printed and bound in Singapore by Tien Wah Press

No professional models were used in the photography for this book.

The material in this book is intended for informational purposes only. None of the suggestions or information is meant in any way to be prescriptive. Any attempt to treat a medical condition should always come under the direction of a competent physician. Neither we nor the publisher can accept responsibility for injuries or illness arising out of a failure by any reader to take medical advice. We are only reporters with a passionate interest in helping ourselves and others maximise potentials for positive health and radiant beauty. This includes being able to live at a high level of energy, creativity and bliss. All are manifestations of harmony within a living organic system and each one plays a vital role in the full expression of the unique authentic power of every woman.

Leslie & Susannah Kenton
South Island, New Zealand 2005

Contents

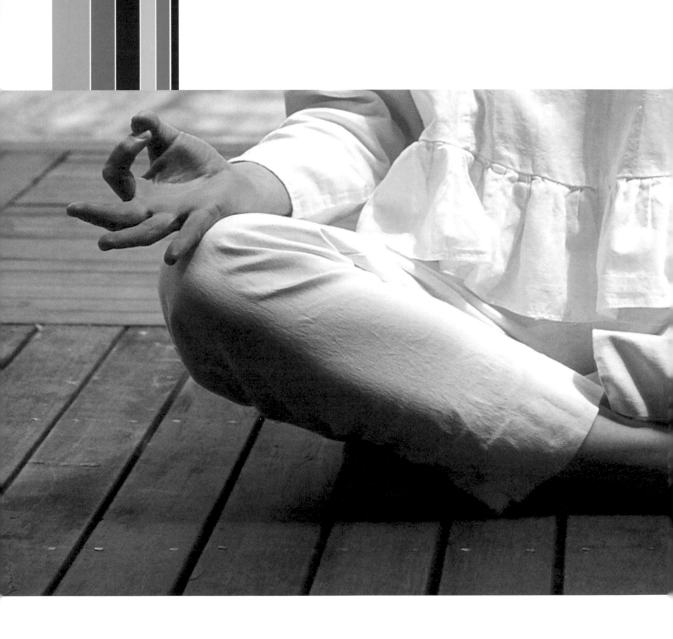

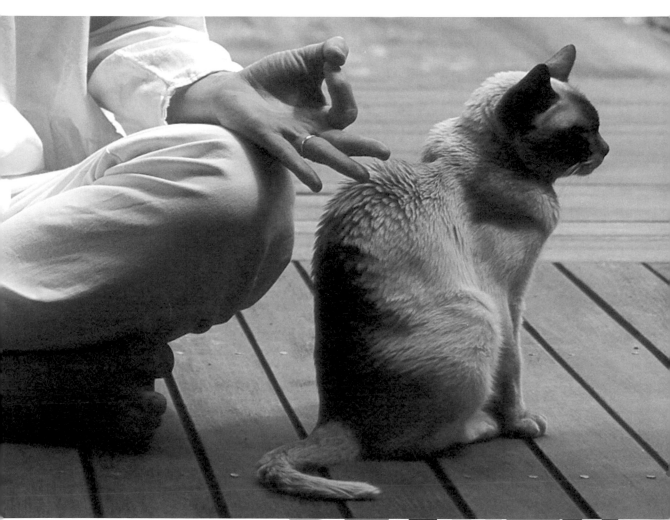

BEAUTY

1 WOMAN REBORN
walk your authentic path

Authentic woman radiates. She's discovered the secret of living from her core. Her world is full of fun, energy and the satisfaction of creating the life she wants. She honours her own truth even when it contradicts received opinion. She dares to be who she is − from the clothes she wears to the work she does. As she watches her life expand day by day, *she knows* that she will find her way. In truth, each of us is already an authentic woman. But few of us have yet discovered it. Too often we go through life neither sensing our authentic power nor experiencing the joy and payoffs living from it can bring. We are taught that 'being an adult' means having to compromise all the time.

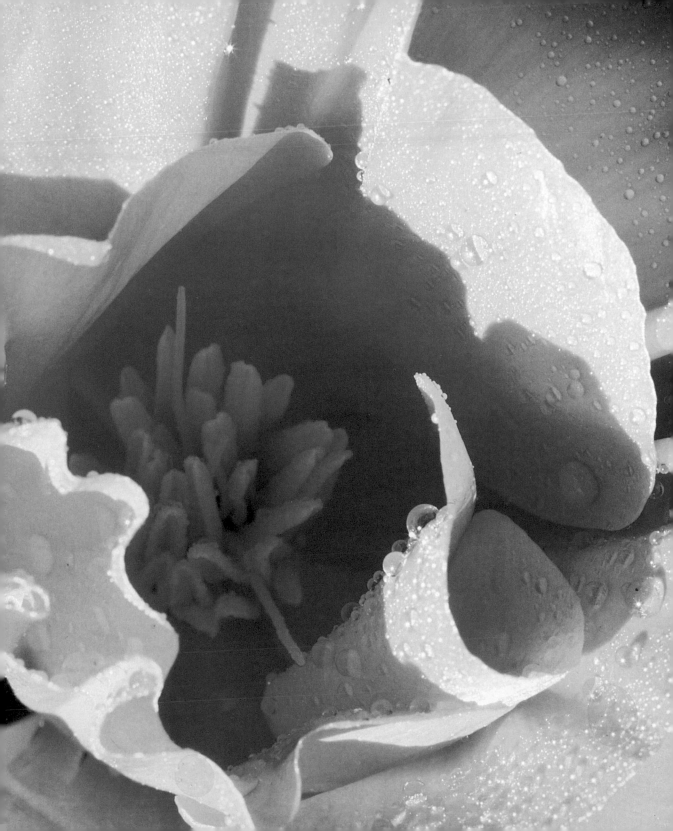

Set Your World on Fire

We alter our behaviour to suit someone, or something, else. We get to the end of the day feeling that we didn't get one thing right – the children didn't eat breakfast, we were late for work, we forgot a nephew's birthday and caused a family rift, we didn't clean the oven and we ate take-away again. To make things worse, we finally fell into bed without doing the hour's yoga/face exercises/meditation we committed ourselves to months ago and haven't done once since. We constantly beat ourselves up. Then we wonder why our lives do not satisfy us. Meanwhile, buried beneath all the noise and bustle that we have gathered around us lies the spark of who we really are. Learn to feed that spark and you can set your world on fire.

BECOME WHAT YOU ARE

Transformation is the name of the authenticity game. Caterpillar into butterfly, base metal into gold as your life becomes an expression of who you are at the deepest levels of your being. Payoffs? Radiant health, good looks, creativity, joy, vitality, relationships that work, fun, a sense of purpose, feeling right in your skin…the list is endless. There's another bonus too: the more you live the truth of who you are, the more those around you – your partner, your friend, your children – become empowered too.

IN YOUR BEST INTEREST

We, Susannah and Leslie, challenged ourselves to gather together all the tools and techniques, information and inspiration fundamental to the process of transformation. Then we asked the question: what combination of these diverse and fascinating discoveries can give a woman of any age the biggest bang for her buck? After all, we live in the quick-fix world of instant coffee and exponentially evolving software, and we expect results.

'You have the power in the present moment to change limiting beliefs and consciously plant the seeds for the future of your choosing. As you change your mind you change your experience.'

Serge Kabili King

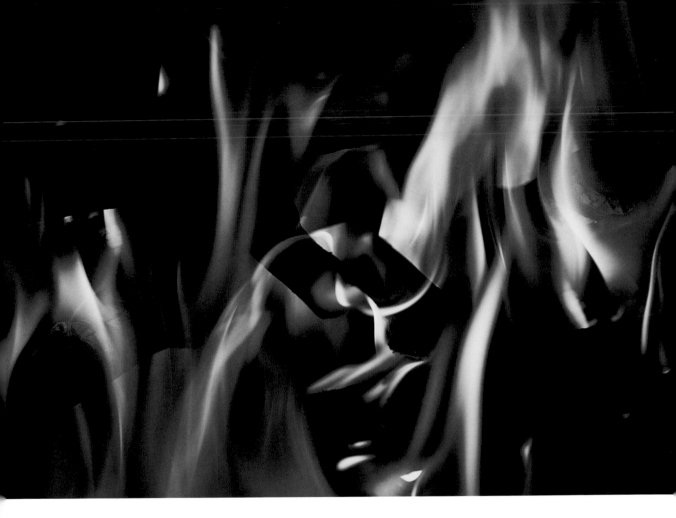

The answer to this question lies in the word *integral*, meaning 'belonging to the whole'. Here we have put together what we believe to be the first integral, ongoing, life-changing approach to beauty, health and creativity for women. It calls on the magic of ancient traditions and marries them with advanced science and consciousness research. Each tool and technique you'll find is designed to work with every other to serve your total process of unfolding. Our intention is to help empower you to become more and more who you truly are. The next challenge is to help you (and us) experience the most fun in the process of transformation. This is how *Authentic Woman* has evolved.

The word 'authentic' means 'genuine, trustworthy, reliable'. It describes a woman who 'acts independently' and is 'author of her own destiny'.

PASSIONATE AND FUN

It's a serious and passionately felt intention. But we ask that you take *lightly* all the techniques, processes and information you find here. Explore with enthusiasm whatever you are drawn to. Never fall into the trap of following blindly what does not ring true for you. And don't treat yourself (or your body) as something that needs 'correcting'. Whenever we do that, bliss and excitement fly out the window and we become submerged in a tedious sea of 'shoulds' and 'shouldn'ts'. If a particular process doesn't grab you, skip it. You can always explore it later. What does inspire you, go for. It can help you change your life for the better – no matter how good (or not-so-good) it seems at the moment.

Try not to let any of the practices you work with turn into obsessions. You don't want to end up with a 'transformation hernia'. Working and playing with this stuff is a game. Approach it with a spirit of adventure. You'll find some of the rewards immediate. Others are more long-term. You might discover a new sense of your own strength or beauty almost instantly, or you may come to realize over several months that your connection with your partner has become deeper and more joy-filled. Each practice you choose to work and play with empowers others, and in turn, the whole of you. That is what integral transformation is all about. It is very much like cross-training.

CROSS-TRAINING

Top coaches make their athletes do cross-training for peak performance: an athlete trains in two or more practices in addition to his or her main sport – almost always unrelated to it. A swimmer might do resistance training and yoga or practise gymnastics, for instance. This helps develop a wide variety of physiological, neurological and mental skills and interconnections, all of which contribute to the process of integration that builds top performance in the athlete's chosen sport. *Authentic Woman* offers whole-woman cross-training for body and soul.

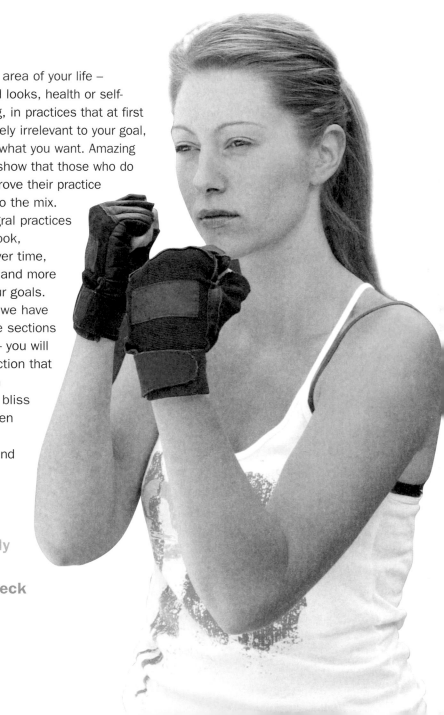

If you want to excel in any area of your life – relationships, career, good looks, health or self-confidence – cross-training, in practices that at first glance may seem completely irrelevant to your goal, empowers you to achieve what you want. Amazing though it seems, studies show that those who do Vipassana meditation improve their practice by adding weight training to the mix. In the same way, the integral practices you are drawn to in this book, successfully carried out over time, can help you realize more and more of your wholeness and your goals. This is also why, although we have divided the book into three sections – Beauty, Body and Bliss – you will find information in one section that you might expect to find in another. Beauty, body and bliss are integral, so tightly woven together it is impossible to separate them. Find one, and you support all three.

'You cannot avoid paradise, you can only avoid seeing it.'
Charlotte Joko Beck

FROM DISSATISFACTION INTO POWER

When it comes to personal transformation, dissatisfaction – even misery – is often a real blessing. It can fuel the process of transformation. When any kind of suffering brings you to the point where you know something is missing in your life and you want more – more energy, more strength, more clarity, whatever – then you are truly ripe for positive change. Suffering can awaken a desire to realize your highest potentials.

Each of us has access to multiple levels of awareness, strength and energy which we can call on to help realize our potentials. Instead of using them in our favour, too often they get used against us. We spend time disapproving of who and what we are. Want to move out of self-criticism or impossibility into a place of power? Effective integral transformative practices get the job done.

INTEGRAL PAYOFFS

Does authenticity really matter? You bet. The payoffs are so voluminous it's impossible to list them all. You can:

- Live fearlessly.
- Feel fully alive.
- Develop your own unique charisma.
- Live a rich multi-dimensional life.
- Become ageless.
- Be free to tell the truth and be what you are.
- Live spontaneously.
- Make choices from freedom, not fear.
- Live with greater ease and grace.
- Care for yourself at least as well as you care for others.
- Have a hell of a good time.

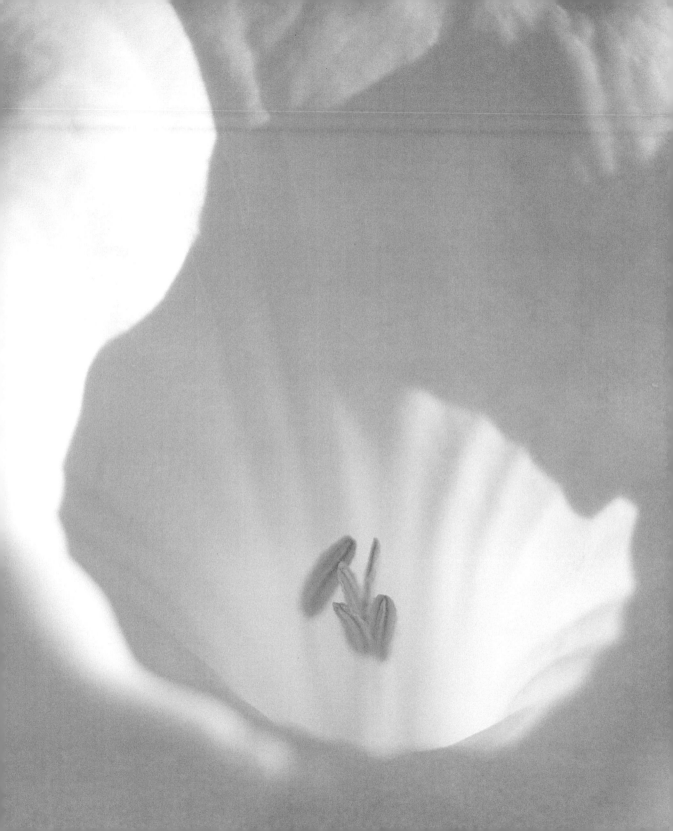

AUTHENTIC WOMAN'S JOURNAL

Throughout the book we ask you to use a Journal to record thoughts, feelings and revelations, and to work and play through various processes. This is no ordinary journal where you write about what you did that day. It is a place for you to map out your personal path to authenticity step- by- step. Your Journal bears witness to the unique process of your own unfolding. Short of being able to take you through each exercise and process in a workshop setting, and hear your feedback and discoveries in person, it makes it possible for us to work as intimately as possible. It also helps you get to know yourself at the deepest level and celebrate who you are, with abandon.

You can rediscover your own authenticity, celebrate it, immerse yourself in the beauty of who you are, reawaken the life in your body, rekindle the creativity that is your birthright and live a life that feels supported and rewarding on every level. Sounds too good to be true? Then you may not, as yet, have fully tapped the richness at the core of your being – that divine spark that makes you unique in every way yet which paradoxically connects you with all of life.

To write this book we have had to learn to *live* it ourselves. It is not about theory but about practice, discovery and the excitement that grows week by week as more of you becomes present to play the central role in your life unfolding.

'Where there is great love there are always miracles.'
Willa Cather

The pathway to authenticity is more than a journey, it is an immersion in a way of feeling and thinking, living and dreaming that to many of us seems brand new. Yet within the newness, most women find ancient echoes of something long forgotten which, at the deepest levels of our awareness, we have in truth never forgotten at all. It's like diving deep into a lake where the water is shot through with streams of light in constant motion – now gentle and lulling, then wild and filled with the exhilaration of wind or the pounding of rain. It's like coming alive.

CALL TO ACTION

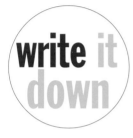

Get A Journal: If you already have a journal you love to write in, great. If not, treat yourself to one soon. It should be special. Make sure it is large enough that you don't feel cramped writing in it. Find a cover that inspires you. Or draw, paint or make a collage for the front of it. This is a place where you will explore a new relationship with yourself and your life. Whatever you do, don't settle for anything less than the very best.

Make Your Mark: Open your journal and make your mark on the first page – any mark at all. Simply write your name with your favourite pen. Or draw a picture, write out the words of an inspirational song or poem, or write down a few of the things that are important to you right now. Make the journal your own.

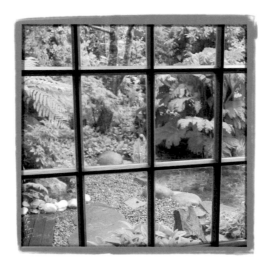

'Things do not change –
we change them.'
Henry David Thoreau

2 BEAUTYFEST
indulge your senses

Narcissism? No way. Authentic beauty is generous, all-encompassing and a delight to behold. It is born out of self-actualization, not self-obsession. Discernment, self-respect, savvy and playfulness — these are its watchwords. Authentic beauty is not just holistic. It is *integral* and powerfully transforming. Get ready to adorn yourself as never before. Colour, texture and fragrance can shift your moods, delight your senses and awaken your full potential for self-expression. Let the clothes, jewellery and scents you wear and the energy you create around you, transform how you feel about yourself, relate to others and live your life.

INTEGRAL BEAUTY

Authentic beauty doesn't stop at the cream you use or even at the edges of your body. It encompasses sensuous products and practices, counters stress, heightens vitality and brings a sense of personal freedom. Everything you choose for adornment – from an aura spray based on the energy of top-grade essential oils, to a pair of red shoes, fresh flowers, and scented candles – is all part of the process. It can enhance the whole of you.

Dress To Kill Convention

A couple of things inhibit the creativity and fun you can have with clothes. The first is negative beliefs about your body. The second is limiting assumptions about what suits you or what you're *supposed* to wear. Why not suspend your judgments for a while? Is there a seductress hidden beneath your intelligence and efficiency? A 'romantic' longing for expression? A latent businesswoman dying to shed those sweat pants and step out in a power suit? Let's find out.

WHAT CRAMPS YOUR STYLE?

In your Journal, make a list of all of the things you believe are holding you back from dressing the way you'd love to. What are your style crampers? For instance:

- I'm overweight.
- My breasts are too big/too small.
- I can't wear a skirt because of my varicose veins.
- I can't afford nice clothes.
- I'm too short/tall.

Now take a good look at what you've written and ask yourself if what you believe about yourself is really true. It's easy to mistake beliefs for truths and feel imprisoned by them. For instance, is it true that overweight/very tall or very short women cannot look great in clothes? Hardly. Is it really true that you can't afford nice things? What about second-hand shops, swapping clothes with friends or even making your own? Which of your beliefs might you be willing to loosen your grip on to expand your potential for fun in the dress-up department

'A fashion is nothing but an induced epidemic.'
George Bernard Shaw

The woman caught sight of her reflection in the mirror and stood transfixed, as if seeing herself for the first time: she marvelled at the blue lace network of veins across her chest. She noticed the stretch marks across her belly and began to smooth them with her fingers, remembering the magic of the twins' birth and the delight they brought her daily. She began to smile. As she did, she saw how deeply etched the lines around her eyes and mouth had become. She was a woman who had laughed too loud, too often. She was indeed blessed.

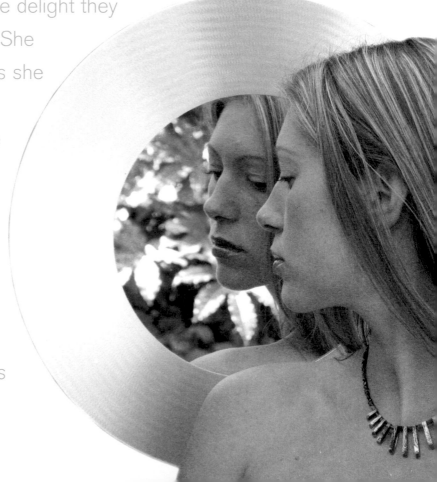

YOUR PASSION STATEMENT

Defining your style means letting passion guide your clothing choices rather than someone else's idea of what's in. Create your passion statement by drawing inspiration from things you love. Take out your Journal and explore the following:

> **Name a type of animal or bird that you love. What quality do you appreciate most about it? Example: Dolphin – playfulness.**

> **Think of an actress in a film you love. Which of her character's qualities do you appreciate?** Example: Grace Kelly in *High Society* – elegance and carefree abandon.

> **Name a flower you love. What quality does it represent to you? Example: Peony – opulence.**

> **Think of a person (man, woman or child) whom you love and admire. Which of their qualities do you appreciate most? Example: My friend Lance – adventurous, a risk taker, practical.**

> **Think of a landscape that you love. Which of its qualities appeal to you?** Example: A pine forest – clean, uplifting.

In your Journal, circle the qualities you've identified, then use whichever feel appropriate to create a passion statement:

> For example: My style is playful, elegant, carefree, opulent, adventurous, practical and clean.

Write this statement out and post it on your wardrobe. Keep it in mind when you shop for clothes. It can help guide you to make choices in keeping with your passion and authenticity.

After making your passion statement, and clearing out beliefs that inhibit your style, go to work on your wardrobe. Get rid of anything that doesn't bring you pleasure or support your authentic expression. Use the Wardrobe Overhaul exercise below as a quantum leap into authentic living.

> 'I wish I had invented blue jeans. They have expression, modesty, sex appeal, simplicity – all I hope for in my clothes.'
>
> **Yves Saint Laurent**

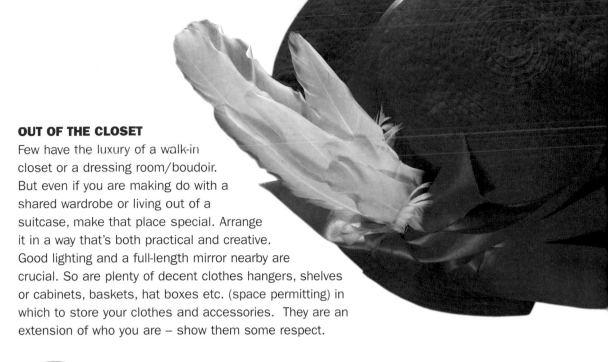

OUT OF THE CLOSET

Few have the luxury of a walk-in closet or a dressing room/boudoir. But even if you are making do with a shared wardrobe or living out of a suitcase, make that place special. Arrange it in a way that's both practical and creative. Good lighting and a full-length mirror nearby are crucial. So are plenty of decent clothes hangers, shelves or cabinets, baskets, hat boxes etc. (space permitting) in which to store your clothes and accessories. They are an extension of who you are – show them some respect.

wardrobe overhaul

Go through your whole wardrobe. Remove anything you don't love or haven't worn for a year. 'File it' in one of two piles:

The 'gotta go' pile:
● It's worn out, stained or damaged beyond repair.
● It doesn't fit and never will.
● It's too uncomfortable/itchy.
● It makes me feel 'less than' when I wear it.

Once you have created your 'Gotta Go' pile, see which pieces someone else might like and donate them to charity. Put the rest in a clothes recycling bin.

The 'needs help' pile:
● Anything that you might wear if it were dry-cleaned, repaired, altered, dyed.
● Things that you would wear if you had something to go with them.

Now take action with the clothes in this pile. Get things fixed, find/buy coordinating pieces, or add them to the 'Gotta Go' pile.

Once you've cleared out what you no longer want, reorganize your wardrobe in whatever way suits you best. This process can bring order to thoughts and feelings as well as clothes. You might like to arrange clothing according to modes – work mode, fun mode, lounging mode, or dress-up mode, for instance. Or maybe by colour. Go with whatever inspires you.

Smart Shopping

Time to consider the gaps in your wardrobe. What's missing that you would love to have? It could be casual, smart, dressy, sporty, wild, comforting, nostalgic – whatever. Make a wish list. Pledge to fulfil it over the coming weeks and months. Instead of getting sucked into a shopping frenzy that leaves you feeling like you need a good shower inside and out, be deliberate in what you look for. You might take a friend along whose taste you admire, or even treat yourself to a personal shopper whose expertise could open your eyes to new possibilities. Above all, opt for clothes that really make you look and feel great. Go for fabrics and colours that delight your senses – including textures like silk or cashmere that caress your skin. Choose outfits that make you come alive. Turn shopping into an integral experience.

'If you never have, you should. These things are fun and fun is good.'

Dr Seuss

GO COLOUR CRAZY

A couple of years ago, on the way to give a talk at a beauty conference, we were met at the airport by a lady who was a colour consultant. We had a couple of hours to spare, so we asked her to 'do our colours' – something we had always secretly thought was a waste of time. It was an enlightening experience. We took to heart much of what she shared with us and laughed a lot about Leslie with her passionate nature being typed as a 'Light Spring'. We discarded a few fascist statements like, 'Leslie, from now on navy is your black', but it opened our eyes to many great colours we would never have considered wearing before. (Needless to say, Leslie has not forsaken her beloved black.)

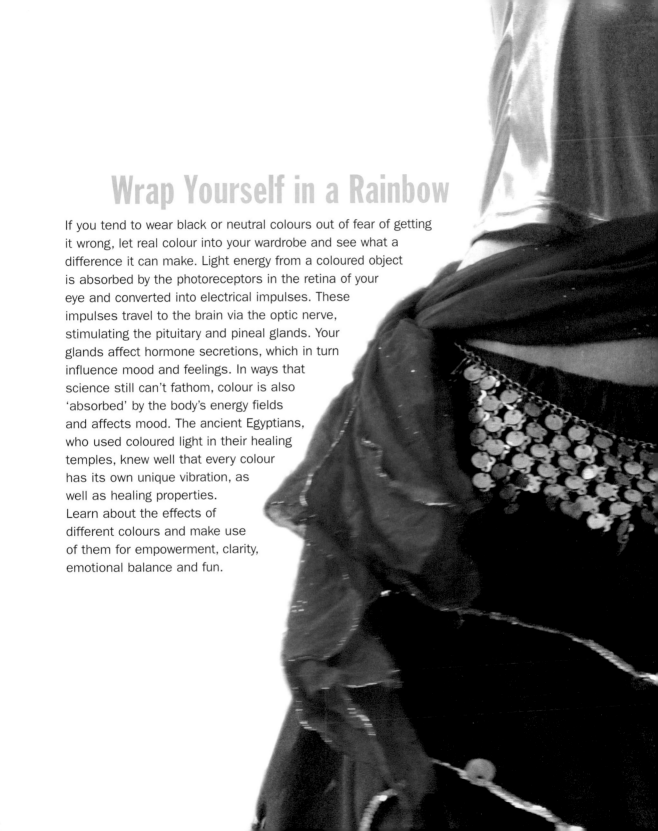

Wrap Yourself in a Rainbow

If you tend to wear black or neutral colours out of fear of getting it wrong, let real colour into your wardrobe and see what a difference it can make. Light energy from a coloured object is absorbed by the photoreceptors in the retina of your eye and converted into electrical impulses. These impulses travel to the brain via the optic nerve, stimulating the pituitary and pineal glands. Your glands affect hormone secretions, which in turn influence mood and feelings. In ways that science still can't fathom, colour is also 'absorbed' by the body's energy fields and affects mood. The ancient Egyptians, who used coloured light in their healing temples, knew well that every colour has its own unique vibration, as well as healing properties. Learn about the effects of different colours and make use of them for empowerment, clarity, emotional balance and fun.

COLOUR YOURSELF BEAUTIFUL

● **Red** stimulates. It increases heart rate, circulation and brain activity. The colour of passion, power and desire, wear red to feel strong and energetic.

● **Pink** is soothing and calming. It relaxes muscles and subdues aggression. Wear pink to uplift when you feel discouraged. Peachy tones are good if you feel emotionally depleted.

● **Orange** strengthens the immune system and is good for digestion. A cheerful, warming, grounding colour, orange boosts self-esteem, clears inhibitions and promotes enthusiasm for life.

● Yellow supports your nervous system. It can help you make decisions and feel alert. It is uplifting and mentally stimulating. Wear yellow to encourage optimism and rational thoughts.

● Gold carries power for transmutation and abundance. It symbolizes divine perfection, spiritual awareness and wisdom. Wear gold to strengthen your energy fields.

● Green helps to balance the emotions and calm the nerves. It is the colour associated with heart energy. Wear green or turquoise to promote serenity and peace.

● **Blue** lowers blood pressure and slows heart rate and respiration. A cool and soothing colour, it connects you with intuition and supports clear communication.

● **Purple** encourages spiritual awareness and access to subtle realms of consciousness. Wear purple to connect with your ideals. Reddish purple is more energizing. Indigo and lavender are more calming.

● White cleanses and purifies the spirit and emotions. It is the colour of peace. Wear white for centring and protection from stress caused by too much sensory input.

● **Black** connects you with the mystery of the feminine. It is the colour of the void. Wear black when you want to enhance introspection.

● **Brown** is grounding and stabilizing. The colour of the earth, brown is reassuring. Wear brown to ground you, but not too much of it or you may feel depressed.

ARE YOU A RETAIL ZOMBIE?

In clothing shops – especially those in large shopping centres – it can be hard to stay conscious as you shop. Recycled air thick with positive ions (the bad guys), muzak and bored or overly keen sales assistants, can leave you feeling drugged and unable to make the kind of choices that honour you. If you find yourself in this state often, keep shopping trips short and to the point. Refuse to be swept into retail addict mode or to be convinced to buy things you don't want or need. Keep it simple and fun.

Aspirational Scents

Fragrance, like clothing, makeup and colour, is another wonderful way to explore the nature of your authenticity. Most women choose perfume not as an expression of their personality, but as a quality they aspire to. A sexually assured and outgoing businesswoman may go for a delicate floral. Her shy and introverted sister may opt for a seductive oriental. Experiment with fragrance from the various perfume categories to help reveal an aspect of your authentic self.

Orientals: For the would-be Femme Fatale or Wild Woman.

Greens: To call forth the Adventurer or Cool Intellectual.

Florals: To express the Sensual Romantic or Dreamer within.

Aldehydics: For the Power Player or Sophisticated Lady.

If you are not familiar with these perfume categories, ask a shop assistant for help. You needn't limit yourself to one fragrance. Create a perfume 'wardrobe' with scents to match every facet of you. Don't let brand-name snobbery or advertising sway you in your choice of fragrance. Don't even let gender stand in the way of trying men's fragrance if you choose. Let your nose and your intuition be your guides.

When shopping for perfume, here are a few things to consider:

- **Strip Test:** Try perfume on tester strips first. Don't put anything on your skin until you're sure you like it.
- **Sniff Lightly:** Your olfactory receptors tire easily. Don't overwhelm them by trying more than a handful of fragrances at one time.
- **Coffee Break:** Take a few coffee beans in your pocket and sniff them between scents to 'clear your palate'.
- **Long-Term Affair:** When you find a fragrance you like, don't buy it immediately. Instead, spray it on and walk about for an hour or so to let the perfume develop. If you still like it as the middle and base notes unfurl – go for it.

SERGE'S SCENTS

We are both great fans of the perfumes of Serge Lutens. They are made from some of the finest essences in the world. 'Sa Majesté La Rose' is particularly exquisite. It's the best rose we've found anywhere. So too are some of the fragrances available exclusively at Lutens' wonderfully quirky Les Salons du Palais Royale boutique in Paris.

MAKE YOUR OWN

Don't rule out using good-quality pure essential oils to fragrance your hair and body. Relatively inexpensive, they can be combined to create your own unique signature scent. You'll need to dilute them since some can burn the skin if applied neat. Use 25ml each of pure alcohol (vodka will do) and apricot oil with 12 to 15 drops of essential oils. Store your scent in a beautiful perfume bottle and enjoy.

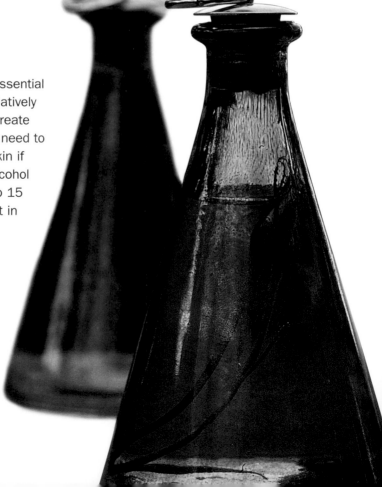

SOUL FEST

When it comes to adorning your spirit, your feelings and your mood, there is nothing like Kate Rossetto's 'Take Me There Mists'. These little bottles are filled with vibrational energies of unique power and pleasure. Leslie keeps several on her dressing table. They can induce sleep, counter the stress of urban life or even help free you from addiction. These fine sprays vibrate with delicate, rich fragrances and powerful intentions. They are part of Kate's 'Scents of Balance' collection of organic and completely natural health and beauty products, which originate in the high planes desert of Montana. Kate grows a lot of what she uses in her products herself. Her 'Take Me There Mists' are integral, they affect everything from your physical vitality to your mental and emotional states. Water-based, with the tiniest bit of alcohol to hold the frequency of the pure essential oil complexes they contain, these sprays sit proudly on a desk or at the side of a bed or you can carry them in a pocket. They come in six different varieties. Whatever inner changes you feel you need, they can help supply them. Want more confidence? Go for her 'Power and Grace' (Leslie's favourite). Long to let down your hair and make some space in your life? Choose 'Freedom'. Feeling Blue? Counter it with 'Joy'. Kate uses no chemical preservatives. Instead, she packages her products in special dark violet glass to preserve them, the way ancient Egyptians preserved their most precious cosmetics.

BEAUTY UNBRIDLED

Spread beauty everywhere. Bring colour into your home by painting one wall a vivid shade or hanging up a swathe of material rich with colours that delight you. Drape colourful chenille throws across your sofa, pepper your bed with coloured cushions. Create 'soundscapes' by playing music or nature sounds that uplift you. Use scented candles or a perfume burner with essential oils to conjure sensual atmospheres. Make colourful bouquets with flowers and blossoming tree branches. Create a shrine in your home or workplace dedicated to beauty for beauty's sake. In the words of John Keats, 'Beauty is truth, truth beauty.
That is all ye know on Earth, and all ye need to know.'

'Let the beauty we love be what we do.'

Rumi

CALL TO ACTION

Make A Statement: Use the Passion Statement exercise to free your imagination for a new way of dressing.

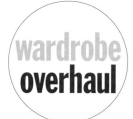

Wardrobe Blitz: Do the Wardrobe Overhaul to give yourself a fresh start and lay the excuse of 'I have nothing to wear' to rest once and for all.

Colour in Action: Use colour to advantage by calling on its healing properties. Want to feel bolder? Wear touches of red – red earrings, red shoes, a red shirt – maybe even consider colouring or highlighting your hair with red. Need to heal a broken heart? Bring more green into your life. Fill your home with houseplants. Want to support your spiritual unfolding? Wrap yourself in a purple pashmina shawl while you meditate.

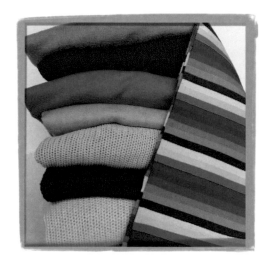

'Use the light that dwells
within you to regain your natural
clarity of sight.'
Lao Tzu

3 FACE YOUR BEAUTY
and live it

Discover and define your authentic beauty. It's an exciting process. If you look in the mirror and don't yet see beauty, be patient. We'll help you call it forth through playful processes and rituals, empowering dietary change and well-chosen make-up. Our goal? To reveal the radiance that is your birthright.

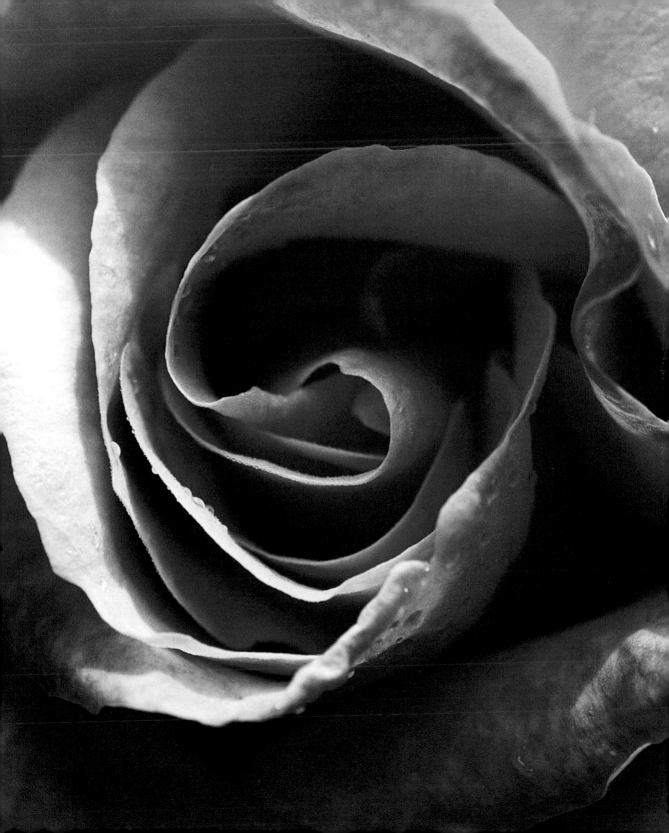

With New Eyes

'There is no excellent beauty that hath not some strangeness in the proportion.' **Francis Bacon**

TRY THIS: Imagine you have a companion who has just come to Earth. She is your age, but without your experience. It's your job to care for her with all the love and compassion you would give a child, a best friend or an animal you cherish. She needs a name, so you give her your own with 'San' added at the end, for example 'Kara-San'. (In Japanese the suffix 'San' is a way of showing respect.)

NEXT: Find a mirror. Close your eyes and open your heart. Let your heart be filled to overflowing with love. (You might imagine a beautiful place, a sunset, or a person you love deeply.) Let the love grow until you feel radiance in the centre of your chest. Now open your eyes and meet your new companion '— San' in the mirror. Look at her face from all angles, touch her skin and hair – explore who she is.

NOW: Pick up your Authentic Woman Journal. Make a note of what you see and what you might do to enhance your companion's beauty, using these guidelines:

● **What do you notice that you love about your companion? It could be a physical feature or a quality, such as 'she has pretty teeth' or 'she looks playful'. Write it down.**

● **How would you like to care for her? Would you: Colour her hair or cut it? Treat her to a face mask? Try out a few shades of lip colour to see which suits her best?**

● **Is there action you can take today to honour your companion's beauty? Make a hairdressing appointment? Reshape her eyebrows? Apply lip-gloss? Do it.**

Beauty Check-In: Any time you look in the mirror and find yourself being overly critical – seeing only your wrinkles or a nose you dislike, catch yourself and stop. Then, close your eyes, centre in your heart, reconnect with your companion '— San' and look again. Ask whether there is anything she needs in this moment and see what you can do to provide it. To blossom fully, authentic beauty needs compassion and care, not judgment and criticism. Practise them.

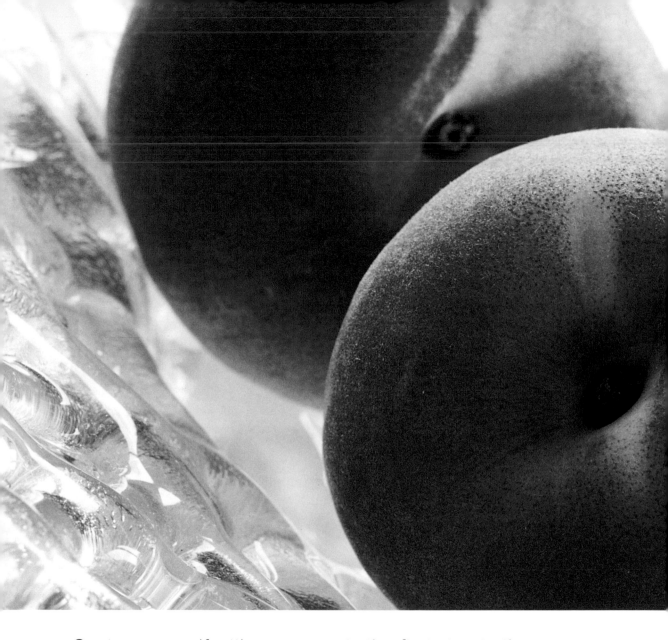

Seeing yourself with new eyes is the first step in the process of living out your authentic beauty. Next, discover how to care for, refine and celebrate your beauty from inside and out.

'Appear as you are, be as you appear.' **Rumi**

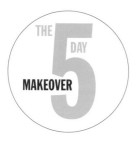

THE 5 DAY MAKEOVER

Radiant, clear skin is a perfect foundation for authentic good looks. If that feels like a distant dream, take heart. In as little as five days you can dramatically improve your skin's look and feel. You may even have friends and family asking which health farm or cosmetic surgeon you've been to.

Inner Face Lift

This little gem of a diet works wonders. We use it ourselves when we want to look and feel our best fast. It lifts, firms and contours skin and softens lines. It brings a glow to your eyes and radiance to your face.

On rising
- 200ml spring or purified water with juice of a lemon squeezed into it

BREAKFAST
- 3/4 cup porridge made with steel cut or rolled oats. Not 'instant oats'. They shunt too much sugar into your bloodstream too fast.
- 1 grated or chopped apple or a handful of berries (strawberries, blueberries, raspberries, loganberries, blackberries – fresh or frozen)
- 1 – 2 tablespoons walnuts – preferably chopped but whole is OK (optional)
- 1 – 2 tablespoons almonds – preferably chopped (optional)
- 1 tablespoon cold-pressed flaxseed oil added after the porridge has been removed from the stove
- A dash of cinnamon (optional)
- 1 cup of green tea, ginger and lemon tea (see below) or 200ml of spring or purified water

Every hour or two
- 200ml spring or purified water or a cup of ginger and lemon tea

LUNCH
- Radiance Salad – an inspiring medley of brightly coloured crunchy vegetables (see opposite) dressed with extra virgin olive oil and fresh lemon juice, garlic, herbs and seasoning. Eat it with…
- 100g to 200g of omega-3-rich fish (wild salmon, tuna – fresh or tinned – mackerel, sardines, herring etc.)
- A slice of melon (any kind but watermelon, which is too high in sugar) or a handful of any kind of berries.
- 1 cup of green tea and/or 200ml of spring or purified water

GINGER AND LEMON TEA

Squeeze the juice of one lemon into a cup. Add 1 teaspoon of finely grated fresh ginger root and either a little stevia or a teaspoon of Manuka honey. Pour hot water over all. Steep for two minutes. An alternative to ginger root is a capful of tincture of ginger from a herbalist (nice because it is simple to use and to take with you). Lemon is detoxifying and helps improve your acid-alkaline balance – important for beautiful skin. Ginger brings the fire element into your body for energy, cleansing and good circulation.

Every hour or two
- 200ml spring or purified water or ginger and lemon tea

DINNER
- 100g to 200g of any kind of fish, organic lamb's liver, tofu or an omelette
- Large mixed green salad with avocado dressed with extra virgin olive oil, flax seed oil, fresh lemon juice or cider/balsamic vinegar, plus herbs and garlic
- A slice of melon (any kind except watermelon which is high in sugar) with a handful of berries – fresh or frozen.
- 1 cup of green tea and/or 200ml of spring or purified water

Evening
- 200ml spring or purified water or ginger and lemon tea

Snacks (optional)
If you want a snack, eat one of the following twice a day either between breakfast and lunch, lunch and dinner or at bedtime:
- 50g chicken or turkey breast
- 1 kiwi fruit or a small pear or apple
- A small handful of macadamias or walnuts
- 200ml spring or purified water

Lunch and dinner are interchangeable.

What could be simpler? If you're at home all day it's a cinch. If not, make your lunch the night before and take it with you. If you eat in restaurants, familiarize yourself with the myriad ingredient possibilities for a Radiance Salad and tell the waiter what you want. Good restaurants are usually happy to oblige.

RADIANCE SALAD
It's easy to prepare a gorgeous, whole-meal salad in under ten minutes.
In Salad Mastery (p.116) we'll show you how.

Space for Renewal

While your skin is renewing itself from inside out, renew your attitudes to caring for yourself. We created the Dressing Table Game more than a decade ago to help women honour and celebrate their beauty. It's had a powerful impact on the lives of many, including our own. We encourage you to try it. It means establishing a place in your home – a 'dressing table' – as a living place of experiment, exploration and celebration of your beauty. Doing so establishes the message that your beauty matters, and allows you to take a new sense of delight in caring for it.

PLAY THE DRESSING TABLE GAME

Choose somewhere you like in your bedroom or bathroom. Ideally the place should have a good source of natural and artificial light (for applying make-up or styling your hair) and be near an electricity socket. Sanctify this space by removing anything unnecessary.

Your Dressing Table If you already have a dressing table you like – great. If not, make one from a table with a stand-up mirror, an upturned orange crate covered with a cloth – even a shelf. In addition to a well-lit mirror, a hand mirror is useful to see the back of your head and different angles of your face.

Style It Gather any objects that inspire you – a lace handkerchief on which to place things, a few pebbles or shells, a candle – whatever you find beautiful. Find a photograph of yourself that you particularly like and frame it to place on your dressing table. If you have a favourite quotation or a picture or postcard that pleases you, add that too.

Organize Your Stuff Find a few baskets or boxes in which to organise your make-up, hair things, face and body care products, jewellery etc. If you lack drawer space you can keep things in boxes of different shapes and sizes. Hatboxes are great for bulky stuff like hair accessories. Arrange items so they are easily accessible and fun to use.

Junk the Junk Sort through your beauty things and get rid of everything that isn't useful and doesn't inspire you. If you can't bring yourself to throw something away – like a piece of jewellery you never wear – put it in a cupboard. Your dressing table should hold only the things you like best.

As you sort through your belongings make a list of anything you need, such as the right colour blusher, or some tissues instead of the toilet roll you make do with for blotting your lips. Stock up with the missing items as soon as possible.

Take as much time as you need to get your dressing table right. Notice any feelings that arise. One common one is guilt: 'I shouldn't be spending so much time on myself.' 'I can't really justify this when I have so many more important things to do.' Whatever feelings come up, jot them down in your Journal. No matter how guilty you feel or how unjustified, do it anyway! This exercise brings to the surface all sorts of revelations about yourself that have little to do with face creams and lipsticks.

With your dressing table set up, you're ready to dive into the art of authentic make-up.

'Beauty is the purgation of superfluities.'

Michelangelo

Make It Up

The authentic woman uses make-up consciously when she chooses to wear it, to accentuate and celebrate her beauty. She does not live in fear that someone will see her without make-up. Nor does she shy away from it for fear of 'getting it wrong.' She understands the basics, experiments with products and colours that work for her and applies make-up with creativity and a sense of fun.

We both love make-up. During the Health & Beauty Editor years, we had cupboards overflowing with make-up from every cosmetics company to try out and play with. It was a make-up lover's paradise. It gave us a taste for some very beautiful (and often expensive) products that neither of us have ever recovered from. We've also been blessed to meet, work with and learn from some of the world's top make-up artists. Below are a few tips we've picked up on our travels. Use them as a starting point to experiment with make-up as a way to define, enhance and celebrate your own authentic beauty.

A BRUSH WITH HEAVEN

Good brushes make a huge difference, not only to how well you apply make-up, but to how much fun you have doing it. MAC, Jane Iredale, Trish McEvoy and some of the other top ranges offer an intelligent collection of great brushes to help even an amateur with a shaky hand achieve a professional look. Owning a few beautiful brushes makes the make-up ritual a luxurious affair.

'I adore make-up, but when I was Health & Beauty Editor of *Harpers & Queen* magazine I often defied convention and showed up at the office, or at some ritzy cosmetic launch, bare-faced. Wearing make-up should never be an obligation – always a choice. Naked skin has power. Don't be afraid to show it'.   **Leslie**

BRUSHES AND MAKE-UP TOOLS WE FIND USEFUL:

Powder: A large powder brush and/or blunt-ended fat brush, like Jane Iredale's Handi brush.

Blush: A rounded or tapered blusher brush for blusher or bronzing powder.

Eyes: Three types of brushes are helpful: a medium-sized 'all-over' eye shadow brush for the lid, a tapered contouring brush for the eye socket area, and a smaller smudge brush for blending and highlighting.

Eyeliner: An eyeliner brush, like Trish McEvoy's Precision Eye Lining brush or Flat Definer 212 by MAC. These stiff, synthetic brushes enable you to press powdered eyeliner along the lash line for flawless results.

Brows: A small, angled brush, for filling in brows, as well as a regular eyebrow brush, or dry mascara wand, for combing the brows.

Concealer: A concealer brush, such as MAC's Small Concealer Brush 168. This should be made from synthetic bristles so it can be used wet or dry.

Lips: A lip brush for filling in with lip colour or gloss. The retractable kind is convenient.

Tweezers: Slant tweezers are ideal for shaping brows.

Eyelash Curlers: The best ones have a rounded replaceable rubber pad like Shu Uemura's. Clean, exfoliated skin is the best blank canvas for make-up. First apply a moisturizer and lip conditioner. Wait a minute or two for your skin to absorb the moisturizer. Then blot any excess away with a tissue.

LIT FROM BENEATH: Apply a shimmering moisturizer or make-up primer before your base to give skin a luminescent quality.

'When I'm travelling, or working in the theatre, I take a few treasured objects to establish my "dressing table" wherever I am. One of them is a small vase in which I keep fresh flowers on my dressing table – their beauty inspires me to honour my own.'

Susannah

PERFECT FOUNDATION

We are great fans of Jane Iredale's mineral bases. They look and feel great, offer a physical sun block equivalent to an SPF of 17 and are actually *good* for skin. (See pages 209 – 210 for more on the benefits of mineral make-up). If you like a liquid foundation, Iredale's Liquid Minerals is excellent. It comes in a pump container filled with space-age spheres of pigment. You smooth it into skin with the fingertips. We most often use Iredale's powdered mineral bases – Amazing Base and Pure Pressed Base. They give a super-smooth finish.

Apply powdered base by pressing it into the skin in a gentle scrubbing motion with the flat-cut Handi brush. Layer the product until you get the coverage you want. Amazing Base comes as a loose powder and can be blended with a little moisturizer or light facial oil and applied with a fingertip or concealer brush for extra coverage where needed. PurePressed Base comes in a compact – especially convenient for travel.

The Iredale bases cover so well they camouflage most problem areas like dark circles under the eyes, blemishes, red veins etc. For areas that do need extra help, we like MAC's Select Cover-Up and/or YSL's Touche Eclat. Select Cover-Up comes in a tube.You apply it with a concealer brush where needed before applying your base. Touche Eclat comes with its own brush applicator and reflects light beautifully – great for under-eye hollows.

'I'm not bad, I'm just drawn that way.' **Jessica Rabbit**

FRAME YOUR MASTERPIECE

Eyebrows are the frame of your face. A little attention to them can make a world of difference. If your eyebrows are very fair, consider having them dyed a shade or two darker. If they tend to be heavy, you might tweeze them or have them waxed into shape. To define brows with make-up, choose an eyebrow pencil that is close to your natural colour and use it to feather in areas where the hairs tend to be sparse. You can also use an angled eyebrow brush with powdered eyebrow colour to fill in and shape. A tinted brow gel, or a touch of hair gel on an eyebrow brush, helps keep brows tidy.

MINIMALIST EYES

Many women avoid eye make-up for fear of looking garish. It's a shame. As the windows of the soul, eyes deserve to be adorned. The simplest way is to prime your lids with colour that's a little lighter than your skin tone – maybe a soft peach or cream. For mature skin, a cream-based eye shadow works well. You can then add a little mascara to lashes and leave it at that, or take the next step.

HI-DEFINITION EYES

After applying a light primer to lids, use a complementary colour to emphasize the eye contour, such as a soft brown, grey or plum. Work this colour into the crease and blend it over the outer corner of the lid. Finally, use a highlighter, pearl or matt, under the eyebrow, in the inner corner of the eye and in the centre of the eyelid. Blend evenly.

Now use an eyeliner pencil, or a powder or cream eyeliner with your eyeliner brush, to line the upper lid as close to the lashes as possible. Choose a colour such as brown or charcoal. You can use the same colour for the lower lashes, or choose a slightly lighter shade. Depending on the shape of your eyes, they may look best with just the upper lid lined or just the outer corners of the upper and lower lid defined. See what works best for you.

Finally, use an eyelash curler before applying mascara. Brown and aubergine shades are good for lighter complexions, dark brown or black for darker ones.

A favourite emergency trick used by make-up artists around the world as an antidote to swollen, puffy, morning-after eyes is, believe it or not, haemorrhoid cream. Dab a little around your eyes, being carefully not to get any in the eyes and wait a few minutes. You'll be amazed at the result.

'The fruition of beauty is no chance of hit or miss... it is inevitable as life.'
Walt Whitman

INSTANT RADIANCE

Add natural-looking colour to your cheeks by using a large blusher brush to sweep powdered blush across the apple of your cheeks and up towards the temples. Instead of blusher, or in addition, you can dust your cheeks, temples and chin with a little bronzing powder for a healthy glow.

LUSCIOUS LIPS

If your lipstick tends to bleed, prep lips first with lip primer. Next, outline them with a lip pencil that is close to your natural lip colour or complementary to the lip colour you'll be wearing. Fill in with your favourite lipstick, or with the lip pencil, and top with lip-gloss or lip conditioner to keep lips soft and hydrated.

Mist your face with mineral water as a final touch, to soften make-up and give skin a dewy finish.

CALL TO ACTION

Fresh Look: Try the With New Eyes exercise. It takes only minutes and can dramatically transform your self-image. Use your Journal to record what you notice when you look in the mirror and any ways in which your attitude to yourself changes.

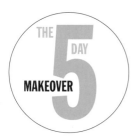

Inner Face Lift: Choose a time when you will try the Inner Face Lift diet. Block out five days in your diary, then make a shopping list of what you'll need and gather the items. Once you discover how much better you look and feel after five days on this program, you'll want to use it often.

Dressing Table Game: Try the Dressing Table Game. Note your discoveries in your Journal. Your dressing table will change as you do. For the process to work best, it needs to remain an on-going exploration of who you are and who you aspire to be.

Play Time: Set aside time to play with make-up. Invite a friend over to share in the fun of it, if you like. Make notes in your Journal: What works for you? What doesn't? What would you like to explore further? What supplies do you need? Playing with make-up (assuming you enjoy it) can help you get to know and express the many facets of who you are.

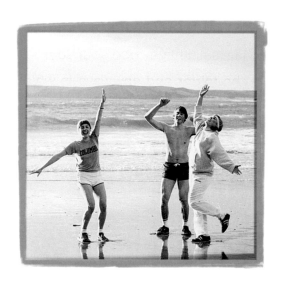

'Youth is happy because it has the ability to see beauty. Anyone who keeps the ability to see beauty never grows old.'

Franz Kafka

4 SOUL FOOD
eat bliss and grow beautiful

Bliss is soul food. It fuels transformation. The human body is the finest resonator for bliss in the universe. Throughout a million years of evolution, our DNA, connective tissue, emotions, energy fields, mind and power centres have been programmed for it. How do you hit the higher octaves of bliss? Expand consciousness, banish limiting beliefs and push the envelope. Become the beauty you already are. There is purpose and wisdom in the pulse of your blood, the flow of your breath, the flicker of an eye. Your body's power and influence, sensitivity and awareness, go far beyond the limits of your skin. Your body – the *whole of your being* – is designed for transformation. Moving through space and time it changes continually. The paradox is that, through all this change, we retain our identity thanks to our inner *core* or *essence* – what is sometimes called the *soul*.

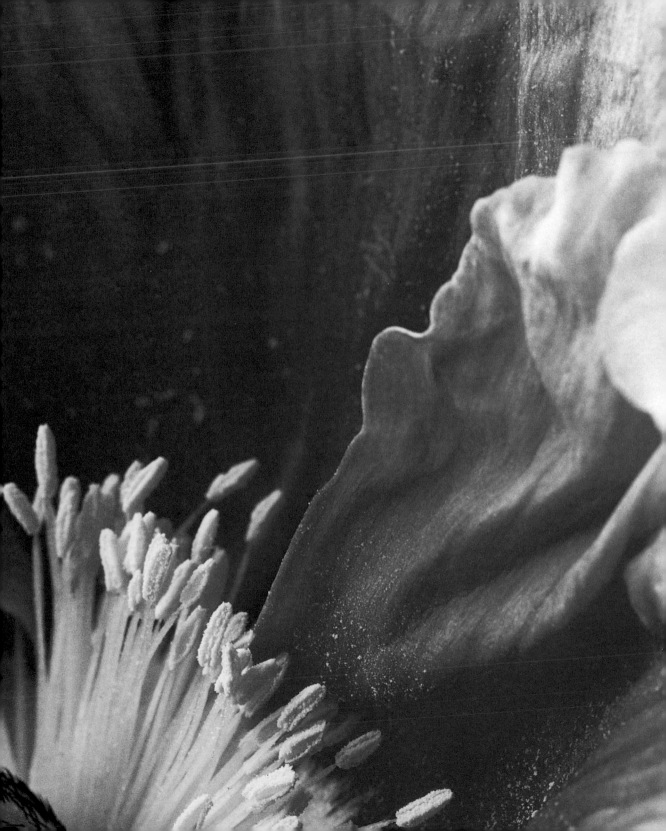

UNIVERSAL POWER

We are literally made out of the same particles of light – photons – that came into being 13.7 billion years ago with the great flaring-forth, the 'Big Bang' that created the universe. You carry within you not only the light energy of the universe but all of its powers: the power to create, to expand, to live in synergy with the rest of creation, to maintain balance, and to transform yourself. In a very real sense, each of us *is* the universe. And, although most of the time we remain unaware of it, our greatest longing is to live out the truth of our essential nature, our core, our soul blueprint – whatever you want to call it – in our day-to-day lives. Honouring this longing puts you on the road to experiencing bliss of the highest order. It is also what makes you authentic.

The reason most women pick up books like this one is they are dissatisfied with themselves – the nose, the hips, the lacklustre hair, whatever. They feel disempowered, not *good enough*. They want to feel better. Trouble is, most advice on how to become more beautiful or more successful or more anything else tells us we need to buy stuff, do something we hate, strive to imitate somebody else or stand back in constant judgement of who we are, how we dress and behave, and the kind of life we lead. Following such advice does not create more bliss in our lives. It does not sort out what we are dissatisfied with. Instead, we have to go to the core of ourselves, find out who we *are* and what we really *want*, then give ourselves permission to have it.

AUTHENTIC POWER

Too many women climb to the top of the ladder to find that it is against the wrong wall. In the process they lose touch with their soul. Authentic freedom and power are never gained by acquiring things from outside. Don't get us wrong. We love beautiful stuff: white linen sheets, fine paintings and delicious food. We love travelling to see the things that fascinate us. But the greatest freedom and bliss has little to do with these things. They come when the part of that iceberg of our own being which lies submerged beneath the sea of mundane consciousness, rises up to greet us with a vision of what is possible, and then provides the energy for us to make it happen.

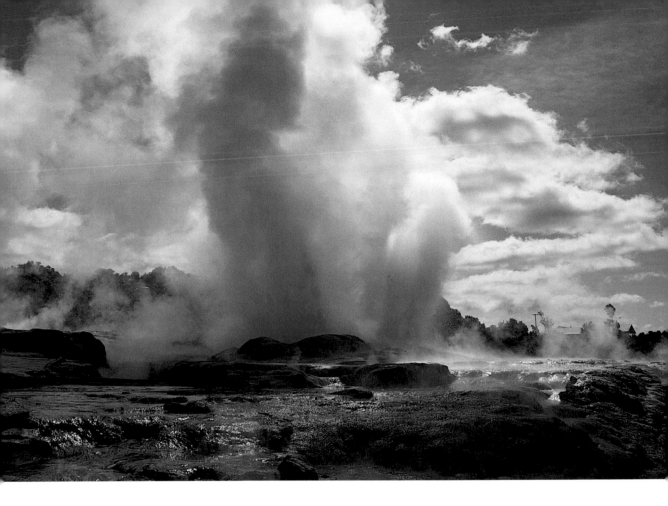

FOUR LETTER WORD

The word 'soul' has sometimes been demeaned, in no small part because of its association with – and *exploitation* by – organized religion. Yet the idea of 'soul' is a familiar one to all cultures – and was so long before Plato put the concept into written words. 'Soul' means the *essential* part or *fundamental nature* of anything – its *animating force* – the seat of personality, intellect, will and emotion, the *inspiring spirit* that both guides and causes movement.

At the heart of every woman, indeed of everything created – dog, flower, rock, the universe itself – is found a singular spirit, an essence, a core, a soul. It carries the physical and spiritual blueprint. Encoded within that blueprint is *intention* which creates who we are and who we are becoming. In every woman, the blueprint is highly individualized. So focused is the energy of intention encoded in your blueprint that it pushes towards fulfilment, reaching towards the light, regardless of what is in its way.

Like the seed of a plant whose genetic material carries the potential for everything it can become as a full-blown tree, each woman carries a package of unrealized potentials for energy, health, beauty, creativity and joy: this physical, psychological and spiritual potential that creates her uniqueness. The more completely she is able to live out her blueprint, the more beauty, power and freedom she experiences.

A woman thrives when she is in touch with her blueprint, when she honours it, and when she makes room for it to express itself in her life. Here's where bliss plays its most important role. Follow what brings you bliss, purpose and meaning and turn away from what does not. The human soul carries a powerful intention to realize fully its unique nature. Following your bliss makes it happen. Like a plant, the soul needs tending for it to blossom.

GENTLE WHISPERS

The soul never *forces* itself into conscious awareness. It waits patiently for you to sense its existence and to welcome it. The soul never sleeps. It whispers to each of us what we need to know to become fulfilled and fully alive. When we cannot hear these whispers or we do not heed them, we become hollow. Life loses meaning. Before long, we become fodder for those who would exploit our misery, telling us that if only we change ourselves, become more reasonable, thinner, better educated, more tractable, buy the latest expensive eyeshadow, then everything will be all right.

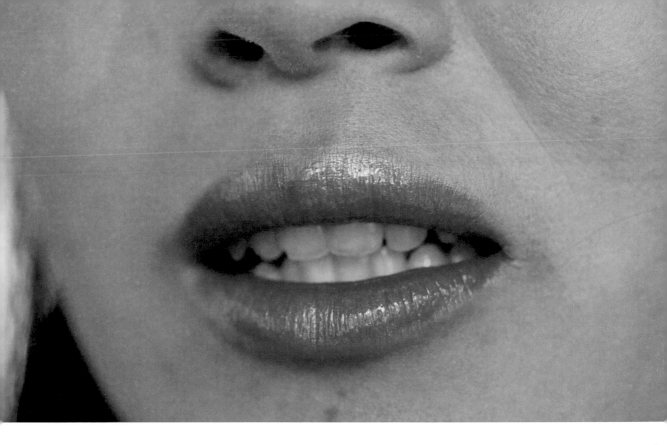

'Our own generation is simply the one to emerge at the time when human consciousness had become subtle enough and complex enough to awaken to what the universe has been telling us from the beginning.'

Brian Swimme

DE-GROOVE YOUR LIFE

To hear the soul's voice, we need to clear away all limiting beliefs about the nature of reality which we unconsciously hold – habitual ways of thinking, moving and feeling. They are like 'grooves' into which we conveniently let ourselves fall for protection from life's surprises. Such grooves can be useful. They bring us structure and a sense of security day to day. After all, none of us can live our whole life standing on top of a cliff while the winds of change toss us about unceasingly.

But our life grooves and limiting worldviews can be soul destroying too. They limit us. They force us to exchange our free, open, positive expectations about what we want to do and be, for distorting self-protective prisons from which we gaze through the bars at what might have been.

BLINKERED HORSES AND MECHANISTS

Our mechanistic worldview is the one we have followed since Newton decided the world was just one big machine. It says that:

- Mind is a function of the physical brain. It has no existence apart from the body and no power to create material reality.
- Intentions, prayers and dreams cannot change the material world.
- The only way we can gain knowledge is through the five senses.
- Phenomena such as ESP, out-of-body and near-death experiences are figments of imagination.
- The universe can be reduced to nothing but an accidental collection of material particles with no purpose and no meaning.

Not only does this out-of-date worldview deny everything we as women instinctively know to be true, it also contradicts every leading-edge scientific discovery made in the last 100 years.

At last, we – especially women – are beginning to turn away from our fascination with *external* power, to replace it with an intention to live our lives with the *creative* power that develops as we build bridges between the inner world of our soul and our outer personality. Such bridge-building creates the foundation for living an authentic life. And our ways of knowing expand beyond the realm of the five senses alone.

SCIENCE MARRIES SOUL

Any blinkered view of reality blocks freedom, entraps creativity, limits bliss and disconnects us, not only from our soul's blueprint and core nature, but from the universe and all its beauty, wonderment and power for growth and transformation.

The *expanded* worldview is called *holism*. It describes the nature of the universe as *holographic*. It is named after the work of scientists who demonstrated that living organisms are integrated energetic systems within an integrated universe. Even our brain and body are holographic. Each part of us, like each part of the universe, is not only connected up with the rest, it embodies the nature of the whole *within* it.

The tension between holism and mechanism – which has developed out of belief in separation between spirit and matter, form and substance – is important to resolve if we are to break out of self-imposed prisons that limit our lives. Be willing to let go of your preconceived notions about what's real in order to explore the further reaches of the newer, wider, more exciting universe. It can be a giant step towards authenticity.

Authentic woman sees past the mechanistic worldview. She demands more space, more accuracy, more possibility. She looks at living systems as integrated wholes. She takes into account the interconnectedness of all things in the universe. Her expanded sense of reality has long been held by mystics from every religious tradition in history. It is an inherently *female* way of looking at life. It honours instinct and intuition, as well as mental clarity and reason. The mystics from every religious tradition insist that we and the universe are *one*. The good news is that such teachings have now crossed over into the realms of science, even though a lot of people haven't figured this out yet. Discoveries in quantum mechanics, systems theory in biology and consciousness research, have blown to smithereens the blinkered-horse view of reality.

'The soul should always stand ajar, ready to welcome the ecstatic experience.'

Emily Dickinson

Expand Your Consciousness

In our ordinary state of awareness we see as though through a veil. We make use of only a very small part of our capacity for creativity, passion, joy and intuition. By *expanding consciousness* we gain access to levels of awareness, experience, insight and creativity generally thought to be only available to artists and mystics. We gain access to our authentic selves. We are not talking about mind-altering drugs or a sinking into uncontrolled states of mind. The best way to explain what we mean is to show you. Try this as a first step in the process of expanding consciousness.

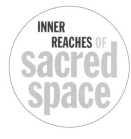

INNER REACHES OF sacred space

This is a process you can use again and again as you work and play your way through the book. Leslie has used it for many years in her workshops. By practising it you will discover your very own sacred place of silence and natural beauty – a sanctuary of absolute safety and a place to which you can return, no matter where you are or in what circumstances you find yourself. Use it for healing, for clarity and guidance, for renewing your physical and mental energy, for cleansing your body or your psyche and for tapping into creativity whenever you wish. This time, your intention is 'to listen to the whispers of my soul'.

Here's how:
- Take the phone off the hook so you won't be disturbed for the next ten minutes.
- Sit on a straight-backed chair, or on the floor if you prefer. Take three or four nice deep breaths through your nose, letting the air escape gently through your mouth on the out-breath.
- Close your eyes.
- Put your imagination into gear. Let your mind go back to some place in nature that you have seen and which you especially like. This is a real place, not somewhere from a dream or a story. It may be a place familiar to you, say, at the end of your garden. Or it can be somewhere you have visited only once.
- When you have found the place you like, sit for a moment quietly remembering as much about it as you can.
- Forget any concerns you may have about your day-to-day life. Allow the wind to carry them high into the sky and far away. Just get in your skin in your sacred place and breathe softly.

● Now see what happens when you activate your senses.

● What do you smell?

● How does the air feel against your skin?

● Sense the earth beneath your body. What is it like?

● What do you see?

● Are there any trees or fruits or flowers around you?

● What do you hear?

● Is there any water there? If so, can you hear it?

● Touch it?

● Drink some of it if you like.

● What does it feel like? Taste like?

● Are there stones nearby? If so, pick one up in your hand and feel the weight of it. Is it rough or smooth?

● What is the atmosphere like? Is the sun shining? Is there mist? Rain? Feel it on your body. Let it penetrate your clothes.

● Let yourself sink into the beauty that surrounds you. In a very real sense this beauty *is* you. All that you see in this special place is part of you and you are part of it.

● Are there any others there with you? Animals? People? Nature spirits? Helpers?

● Let yourself sense the energy of love that surrounds you. It is embedded within your very body by the beauty and the friendship that you take in.

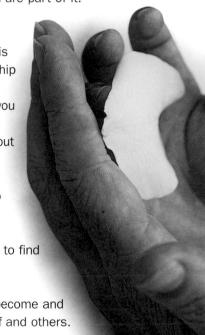

● Simply *allow* the deepest levels of your being to speak to you – in words, in images, in sensations, in feelings. It doesn't matter. You may hear whispers about what delights you, about what you fear, about what you long for.

● When you are ready, give thanks for the friendship and the beauty around you and say goodbye for the moment to your inner sanctuary, knowing that you can return to it whenever you like.

● This place is yours and yours alone. You can come here to find the answer to a question, or for healing, clarity, renewal or refreshment.

● The more often you return the richer the experience will become and the more valuable will be the gifts you bring back for yourself and others.

● Now, very gently, in your own time, open your eyes and come back into the room.

BUILD THE SOUL-BRIDGE

Now take out your Journal and record what you have experienced in the Inner Reaches of Sacred Space exercise. Describe it in words – where you went, what you saw, felt, tasted, sensed, who was there, what happened there, what the whispers of your soul began to say to you. Just let the words flow. Keep writing, without stopping or reading until you have finished. Remember this is not an essay for school. There is no right or wrong way of doing it. If you prefer you can draw what you have seen. This does not have to be a literal drawing, that is of a tree, a flower, a rock. It can simply be colours swirled together to give the feeling of the place or, what Leslie likes best to do, use a combination of words and colours to record your experience. When using colour, the same guidelines apply as for the words, just let rip. You are not trying to be an artist and there is no judgement involved. Let whatever comes onto the page happen. Recording what you experience in your Journal helps to build a bridge between your inner world and your outer one, between your authentic self and the real world.

CONNECT WITH NATURE

Nature is a great carrier of sacred power. Why? Because the energies of nature, in which we have lived as human beings throughout four million years of evolution, are *our* energies. Our bodies and our beings are in communication through our DNA with those of plants and animals. This is what we mean by *holographic*. At a cellular level, we know the familiar taste of herbs and smells of the earth, we are uplifted by the colours of a sunset. This knowing is built right into our being, it is how we connect with who we are.

WHAT ABOUT CONSCIOUSNESS

The Inner Reaches of Sacred Space exercise is a simple introduction to what we mean by the realms of expanded consciousness. Mechanistic science has completely ignored – left out altogether – the power of consciousness. By consciousness we mean not just our everyday sense of awareness, but the vast, multi-sensory realms, rich in creativity, intuition, vision, spiritual experiences, meaning and values. As you have already begun to sense from playing with the exercise, rich inner experience is not only accessible to geniuses and mystics, but to all of us.

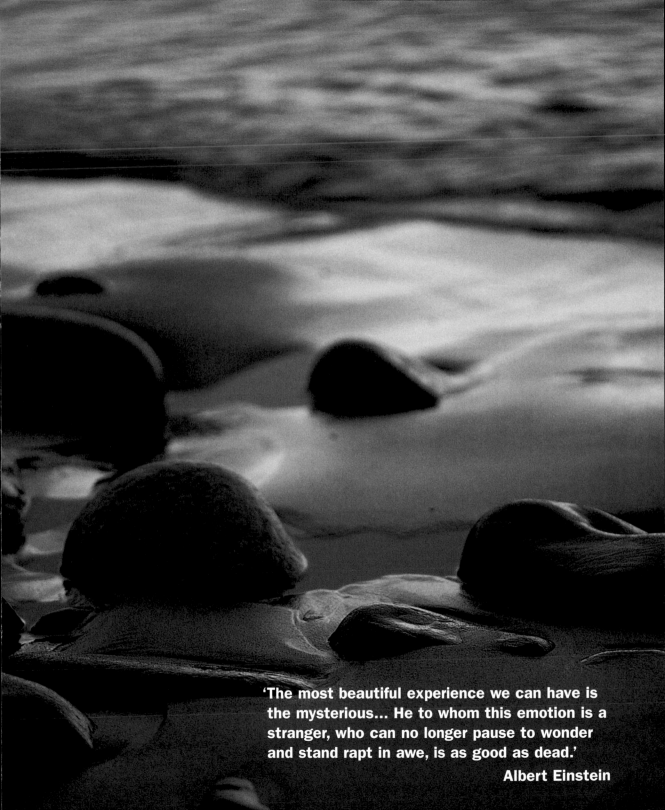

'The most beautiful experience we can have is the mysterious... He to whom this emotion is a stranger, who can no longer pause to wonder and stand rapt in awe, is as good as dead.'

Albert Einstein

Enter the Sacred

The word *sacred* is connected with the sacrum, the lower part of the spine, the 'sacred bone,' valuable above all others. The sacrum defines your centre of physical bliss. It is an inner sanctum of creative and sexual power. *Sacred* is another word tainted by religious overtones. This is a pity, for the process of becoming authentic is indeed sacred in the true sense of the word. It's important to make space for the sacred in your life.

Like our need for bliss, our longing for the sacred is so deeply ingrained in our very being that when we are unable to fulfil it, we end up living in a nihilistic wasteland.

Without a space for the sacred, life becomes narrow, no matter how many fast cars we buy, how many drugs we take, how many lovers we have. Eating, having sex and getting up in the morning become nothing more than physiological events in a mechanical universe. Reawakening an awareness of the sacred opens a door so that each daily routine can, if you so choose, evolve into a 'sacrament' – communion with the sacred. Vitality, beauty and bliss go on and on expanding.

Welcome the sacred. Open the gateway to your own authentic power and freedom. It is difficult. We all knew how to when we were kids. It is just that our educational system, with its emphasis on the rational, the abstract and the pressures of mass conformity has caused us to abandon our intuitive, imaginative abilities. We have been taught to be 'serious', to 'work hard,' not to 'daydream,' 'imagine', or 'be silly'.

Are you finding all this a little deep and sincere? You need only remember what you may have temporarily forgotten and begin to play again. Try this exercise:

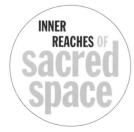

SHOP IN NON-ORDINARY REALITY

Use the Inner Reaches of Sacred Space guidelines. This time, instead of going to your place in nature and asking to hear the whispers of your soul, go to your very own Authentic Woman Boutique. Yes, really. This is retail heaven: the shop assistants are miraculously helpful and knowledgeable and the selection of clothes, shoes, accessories and jewellery is limitless. They always have your size. You never have to go and hang up the clothes you've tried, and everything you want just happens to be on sale. All frivolity aside, using this exercise to explore your personal sense of style and discover clothing that reflects the various facets of your authentic nature can be a liberating experience. Like a childhood game of dressing-up, only better. You can browse to your heart's content or set the intention to find an item for a particular purpose, something to help you feel more confident maybe, or what you'd like to wear at a forthcoming event. The beauty of it is, once you discover things you love in non-ordinary reality – where you are in touch with deeper layers of you – it becomes a lot easier to find the right things in ordinary reality. In effect you are bridging the values of both your inner and outer passion for authentic self-expression.

MYSTERIOUS AND POWERFUL

You can't hold consciousness in your hand or draw a picture. But consciousness has enormous power to affect material reality, something we'll explore further in later chapters. Literally hundreds of researchers throughout the world have carried out well-designed multidisciplinary research as part of what might be called the Human Consciousness Project. Their efforts have converged to form a surprisingly coherent picture of the various states of consciousness available to all of us, and the remarkably rich experiences that can come out of each one. They have also discovered that the blissful realms of expanded awareness – or *non-ordinary* reality such as those you can contact if you continue to work with the Inner Reaches of Sacred Space process – can be mapped just as we can map *ordinary* reality, our day-to-day world.

FREE FROM THE CORE

Our longing for beauty and radiance – to be freely and fully who we are in our core – and our need for bliss, calls us to expand consciousness. It asks us to learn how, at will, both to honour fully our five senses and also to move *beyond* them, becoming *multi-sensory beings*. It asks that we reconnect with our instincts. Instinct, myth, dreams and metaphor are part of the language of the expanded realms. In short, it asks that we come home to ourselves. You can do this without drugs, without gurus, without becoming a disciple of anything or anybody, without having to belong to any privileged group. You can do it regardless of your age, your physical condition or your religious beliefs. The rewards are infinite.

CALL TO ACTION

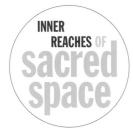

Reach Within: Establish your sanctuary for inner work and explore multidimensional reality with the Inner Reaches of Sacred Space, p.60. Familiarise yourself with the exercise by reading through the instructions several times.

Here is a summary of the steps:

- Journey to your place in nature.
- Activate your five senses.
- Connect with your 'spirit helpers'.
- Ask for help – the answer to a question, for healing, for vitality.
- Give thanks.
- Return to ordinary reality.
- Record your experiences in your Journal.

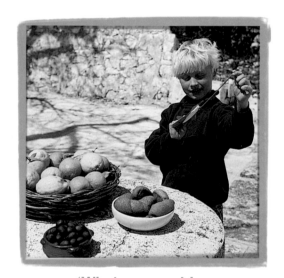

'What we need is
more people who specialise
in the impossible.'
Theodore Roethke

5 INTEND AND CREATE
unleash mind power

The truth is out: mix one part clear intention with a good measure of compassion and you can change material reality. Prayer is powerful. Prayer is an integral practice. When, from a place of stillness, you invoke the power of the universe, nature, helping spirits, God or whatever inspires you, your call brings results. Who says so? A long list of scientists say so, who've done solid research on prayer's effects for healing, for making a dream come true, for living from a place of joy and of freedom.

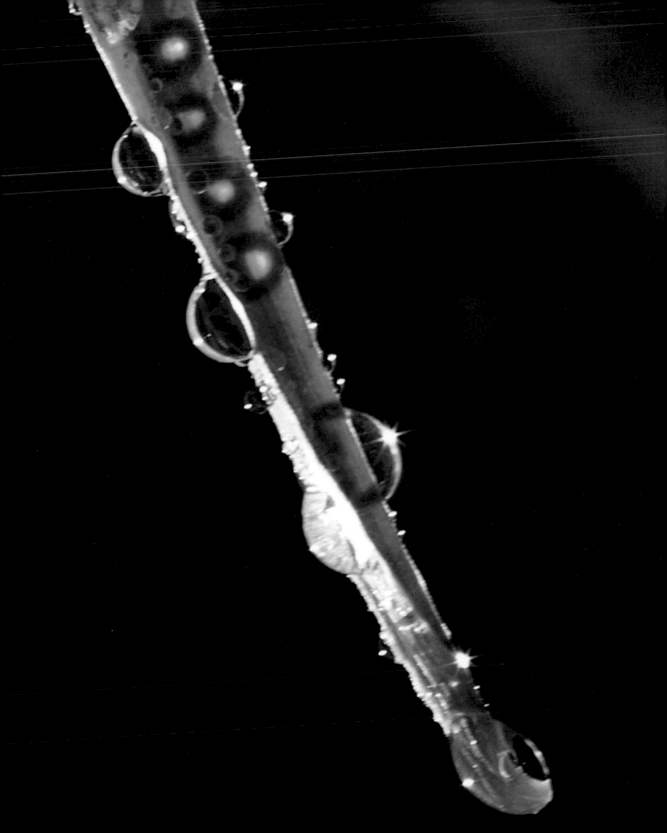

It may surprise you to learn that medical doctors have been so intrigued by what they have witnessed of the power of prayer to aid healing that they have undertaken medical studies on it. It now appears that hundreds of clinical studies have demonstrated that prayer works – even when those prayed for and those sending out the prayers never meet.

At Duke University in the United States, cardiologists Mitchell Krucoff and Susan Craven carried out the MANTRA project, checking out what effects prayer might have on the recovery of heart patients. Neither the patients or doctors knew who was being prayed for. Patients taking part were split into two groups. The names of one group were sent via email to Buddhist prayer groups in Nepal, to Hindus in India, Jews in Jerusalem, Protestant prayer groups and Catholic nuns in the United States, all of whom prayed for them. The other patients were not prayed for. As standard medical treatments for the conditions suffered by these patients produce measurable, expected, side effects, the researchers decided to monitor the effects of prayer on their patients by measuring the side effects experienced. The results were astounding: Heart patients receiving prayer had 50 to 100 per cent fewer side effects from medical treatment.

MIND SHIFTS MATTER

Mind focus changes the reality in measurable ways. Numerous scientific studies have shown that *clear intention* from people in a state of expanded awareness, can inhibit the growth of cancer cells, change the genetic mutations of bacteria, alter the pH of water, shift blood chemistry, increase oxygen levels in cells and even speed wound healing.

Alterations in energy precede physical change. This is a major reason why acupuncture works on humans and animals. When positive energy changes take place, before long the body and mind of a human being can also be changed for the better.

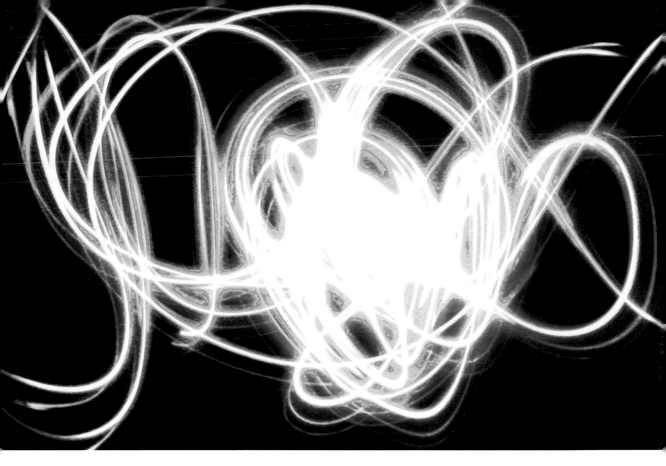

Electromagnetic Changes

We live in a *holographic* universe. Each one of us carries the energy of the entire universe within us. Sincere intention reverberates way beyond us and affects the universe in measurable ways. High level physics has established that a change in one molecule brings about a faster-than-the-speed-of-light alteration to another, even though it's thousands of miles away. This fact has spurred researchers to measure specific *energy* changes in subjects prayed for. In double-blind studies evaluating the impact of distant prayer, American researcher Jack Stucki chose to measure the effects of prayer on human electromagnetic fields. He and his Colorado Springs team checked out electrical activity in the brain and on the body surface of those being prayed for by spiritual groups a thousand miles away in California. Electromagnetic fields in prayed-for people were significantly altered. Those in the non-prayed for group remained unchanged.

'Time and space are modes by which we think and not conditions in which we live.'

Albert Einstein

CHECK OUT YOUR ENERGY FIELDS

Not only are electromagnetic fields altered by thoughts and intention, other complex energy fields surrounding and permeating the human body are also changed. Former NASA scientist Barbara Brennan has created university level training both in the United States and Vienna for enhancing ordinary people's inherent capacity to 'see' or 'sense' these fields. There appear to be at least seven consecutive layers, each of which increases in energy vibration, the further it is from the body. These fields also intersect the body. Thoughts, feelings and intentions influence the harmony and order of the physical body as well as a person's outlook on life, thanks to the powerful effects they have on these fields. Animal studies show clearly that energy fields hold the blueprint for the physical body. Brennan claims the same is true of us.

VISIBLE PROOF

Dr Masaru Emoto, a visionary researcher from Japan, has charted the impact of human consciousness, sounds and words on physical matter in a series of stunning experiments. In 1994, Emoto was studying samples of water from different sources by freezing a few drops and comparing the crystals under a dark-field microscope. Pure spring water shows a beautiful crystalline structure – the beauty of a snowflake. As you might expect, polluted water does not give you a snowflake, it forms a smeary, muddy pattern. What was interesting was that when Emoto exposed water samples to different music, he discovered this can alter the crystals just as surely as pollution in the water. Classical music creates beautiful, harmonious patterns, while heavy-metal music produces distorted, smudged forms. He then decided to take his experiments a step further by writing words on pieces of paper and taping them to clear glass containers filled with water. When Emoto tested the water from the different containers he found that words like 'love' and 'thank you' form delightful crystalline patterns. Negative words and phrases like 'You make me sick' or 'I will kill you' produce muddied, distorted images. After much experimenting, Emoto concluded that the most powerful words and thoughts for creating a high level of order and beauty in the water molecules were 'love' and 'gratitude.' Bearing in mind that the human body, as well as the Earth itself, is largely composed of water, many have come to believe that holding thoughts of love and gratitude, even in the midst of chaos and disintegration, may be a powerful way to promote personal and planetary transformation.

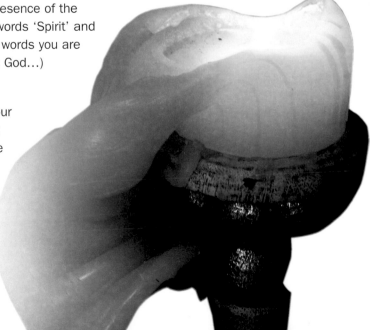

affirmative prayer

Susannah: Affirmative Prayer is one of the most important tools I have ever discovered for harnessing the power of intention to shift reality. Several years ago, I found myself all at once without a job, a home or a car. At the time I was studying Affirmative Prayer in Science of Mind classes at Agape – a non-denominational church in California. I decided to apply what I was learning. Within a month I had found a job, moved into a new home, and been offered a car to borrow for as long as I needed. I've used this form of prayer ever since for healing and manifestation in my own life and the lives of others. You can do it by yourself, speaking the prayer aloud or silently. Or you can share the prayer with another or with a group, letting each person contribute her own affirmations in the 'Realization' stage (see overleaf). It is a great way to discover for yourself just how powerfully your thoughts and intentions create your reality. There are five simple stages to Affirmative Prayer: Recognition, Unity, Realization, Thanksgiving and Release.

Recognition

Begin by opening your heart and mind to the presence of magnificence everywhere and in everything. A great way to do this is to become aware of whatever you love and speak of it. For example: 'I recognize Spirit as rainbows, tree frogs, the hands of a masseur on my body…' Or, simply whatever you notice in the moment, 'I acknowledge Spirit as the birds chirping, the sunlight streaming through my window, the breath that fills my lungs…' Then continue, 'And I know that Spirit is everywhere in everything. There is no place anywhere that the presence of the Divine is not.' (Notice we've used the words 'Spirit' and the 'Divine,' but you can use whatever words you are most comfortable with ? Love, Creator, God…)

Unity

The next stage honours and affirms your oneness with the Divine. So you might say, 'I am one with the presence of the Creator. That which I am, Spirit is, that which Spirit is, I am.'

> 'To fully understand, one
> has to sit down and wait
> for the universe to enter.'
>
> **Brian Swimme**

Realization

In this stage of the prayer you affirm whatever you desire to manifest as if it exists already. This is really important. If you are praying for healing, you might say, 'My body, mind and spirit are perfectly aligned and whole. I experience radiant health on all levels.' You might be battling cancer or dealing with a broken limb, but these are only your life conditions at the moment. The spiritual reality of who you are is the divine perfection of radiant health, wholeness and well-being. Focusing your attention on this truth allows your physical body to come into alignment with it, bringing about the healing you desire.

Words are like seeds planted in the soil of consciousness. Whatever seeds you plant, whatever beliefs you affirm, germinate. This is vital, especially for women, who may feel that they don't deserve health, prosperity, a wonderful relationship, or whatever. The idea of a judgmental God who will only reward you if you are a good girl and who will punish you if you are bad is passé. The creative energy of the universe acts on whatever 'seeds' or thoughts you sow in your mind – consciously or unconsciously. Affirmative prayer helps you choose the seeds you want to grow in your garden – your life.

Thanksgiving

Now give thanks for whatever in your life brings you a feeling of gratitude. Feeling grateful can be likened to shining sunlight and sprinkling water on the seeds you have planted, reinforcing the vibration of your prayer. For example, 'I am grateful for my home and the love of my friends. I give thanks for this opportunity to remember my divine wholeness and well-being through prayer.'

Release

The last stage of the prayer is letting go. Like sighing out, now you surrender your prayer, giving it over fully to the law of the universe and trusting that it is handled. You might say, 'I release my prayer freely and fully into universal law knowing that it is done. And so it is. Amen.'

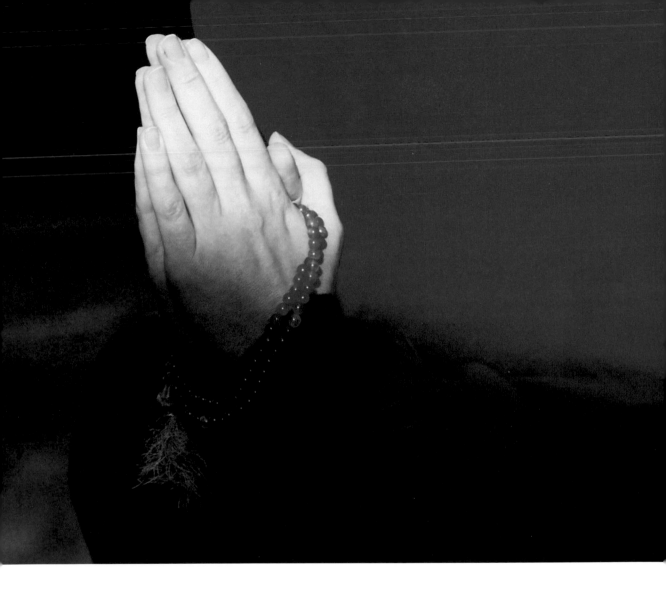

PRAY YOURSELF PREGNANT

A study was conducted at a hospital in Seoul, Korea, during 1998 and 1999 to measure the effect of prayer on fertility. A group of 199 women undergoing in-vitro fertility treatment was divided in two. Half the women were assigned to prayer groups for regular prayer. The other half acted as the control. Neither the women nor the hospital staff knew they were being prayed for. Twice as many of the women who were prayed for became pregnant than the ones who were not.

Parrot Power

A simple tool for invoking the life you want is what we call *intention activator*. It makes use of invocation – a phrase of somewhere between five and ten syllables repeated over and over parrot-fashion and synchronized to your heartbeat. You can work with a single phrase or more than one. We suggest you experiment with one for some time before changing to another. The subconscious, out of which creative power flows, responds more readily to the repetition of a single aspiration. Your invocation repeated over and over becomes a 'tape'. Unlike the negative 'tapes' that unconsciously play in our minds such as 'I could never do that' or 'I am ugly', or 'I am going to fail', the intention activator creates a new positive reality. Repeated again and again, eventually your phrase begins to arise spontaneously. It's like repeating the words of a song. You find yourself waking up to it. You may even hear it in your dreams. In time, your negative tapes become superseded by chosen intentions.

Choose your invocation from the words that mean most to you. They may be words you have already written in your Journal that best describe something you want to create in your life. Here are a few examples:

- I am strong, inspired and at peace.
- I create my world with ease, grace and magnificence.
- Moment by moment I celebrate life.
- I live the happiest, most fulfilling life possible.
- I am clear, creative and free.

Use intention activator while relaxing, meditating, exercising, driving, or going about daily routines. Do it the easy way, without a lot of effort. If you forget to use it for a day or two, don't worry, just pick it up again. Repeat your phrase when you are busy with other things, too, like working, exercising or studying. It can actually contribute to the activity you are engaged in.

'Whether you think you can or whether you think you can't, you're right!'

Henry Ford

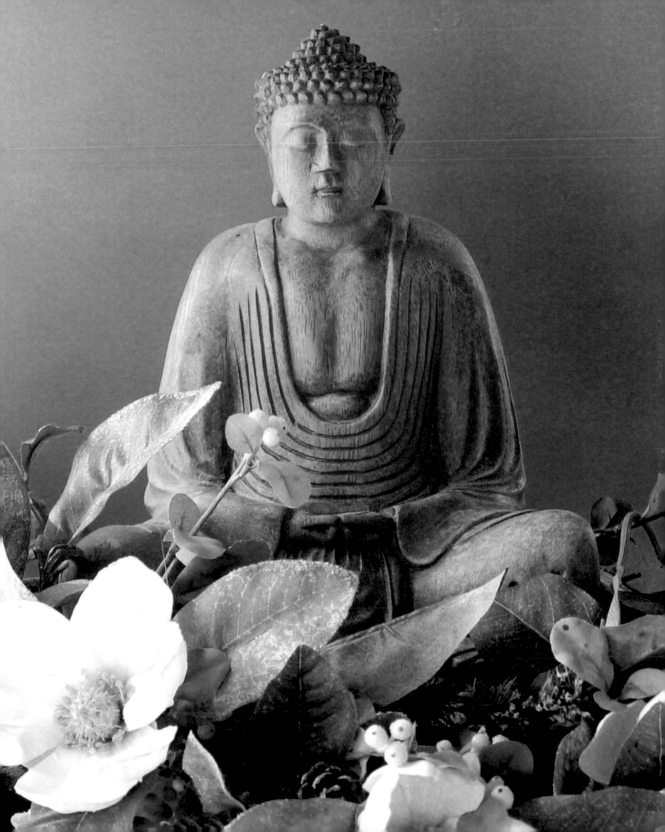

CALL **TO** ACTION

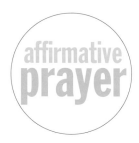

Practise Affirmative Prayer: Explore the power of intention by putting Affirmative Prayer into practice. Whether your prayer requests feel profound or trivial is of no consequence. Don't judge them. Just continue to affirm what you want to create – daily if necessary – until you begin to notice results.

Activate an Intention: Use the Parrot Power exercise to work with the invocation of your choice in any area of your life, such as health, work, relationship, self-confidence, fitness or creativity.

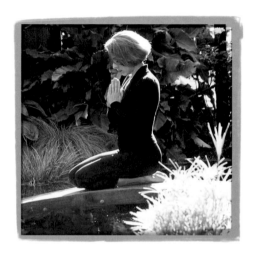

'You yourself, as much as anybody
in the entire universe, deserve
your love and affection.'
Buddha

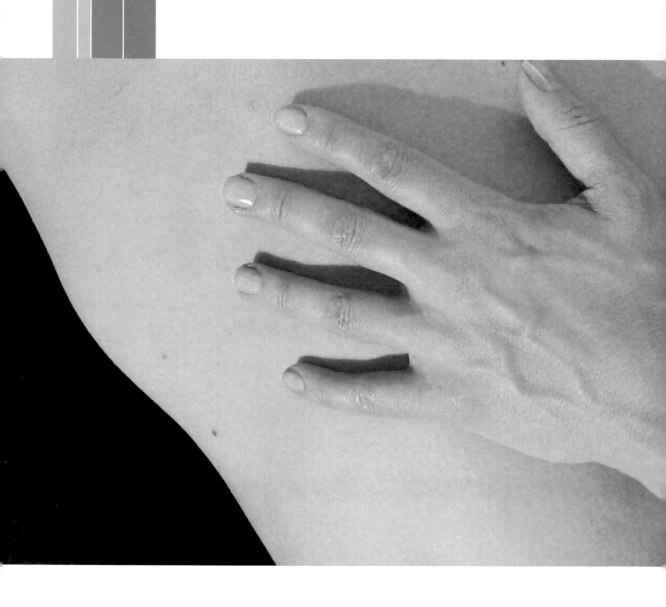

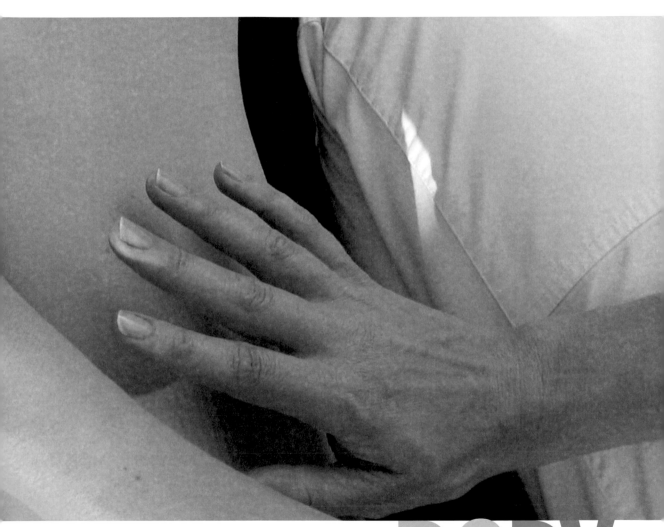

BODY

6 PRIMAL FOOD
eat with the apes

Being authentic means honouring what you need, body, mind and spirit. If you're not eating the foods your body has been genetically programmed to thrive on for more than a million years of evolution, you are really missing out on something.

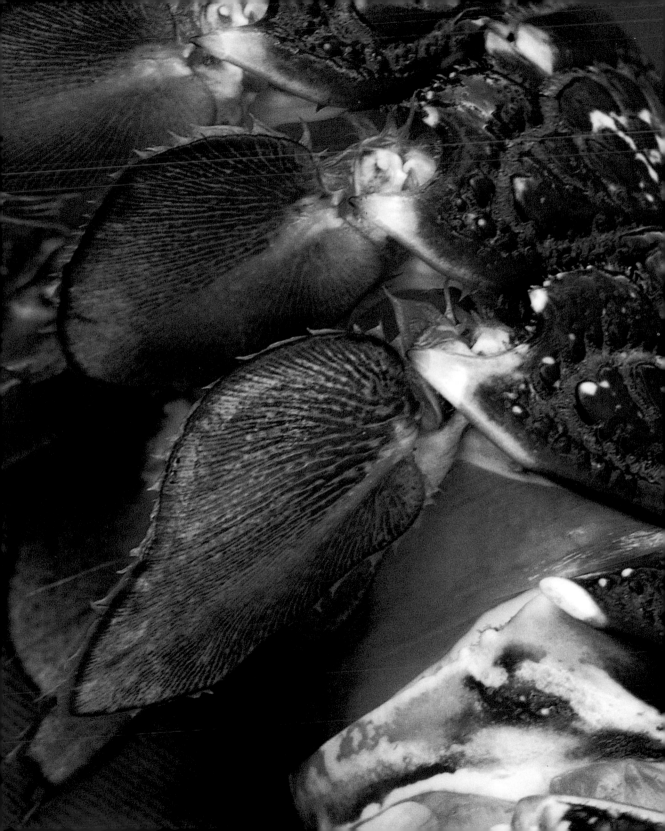

How would you like to discover a way of eating that provides endless vitality, improves athletic performance, helps clear cellulite and PMS, restores emotional balance and enhances mental clarity? Sound too good to be true? A growing number of women take such payoffs for granted. We call them the 'elitists' since they know how to do what the rest are still confused about. From Hollywood stars to top athletes, they have switched to a high-raw, low-grain, protein-powered diet. And they love it.

FOODS THAT CHANGE YOUR LIFE

In the past decade, research findings and clinical experience have combined to create the ultimate way of eating for energy and good looks. We call it *Radiance Eating*. Here's the low-down:

● **Go Palaeo:** Return to an approximation of what our Palaeolithic ancestors ate – top quality proteins plus fresh raw foods. It stops swings in energy and mood, realigns your body to a high level of health, and curbs the development of Syndrome X, the destructive collection of conditions that has now reached epidemic proportions (more about this later).

● **Cut Paste:** Eliminate wheat, maize, flour and anything made from them from your diet, along with sugars, gummy starches and sweets and reduce (or even cut out) other cooked grains. Doing so balances biochemistry, triggers fat loss, restores energy and helps wipe out cravings for alcohol, drugs and sweets.

● **Eat Raw:** Evidence mounts from biochemistry, biophysics and emerging paradigm science that human beings thrive on a high-raw diet of naturally grown foods, thanks both to its vitamin, mineral and trace element content and to the energetic order it imparts to the whole of you.

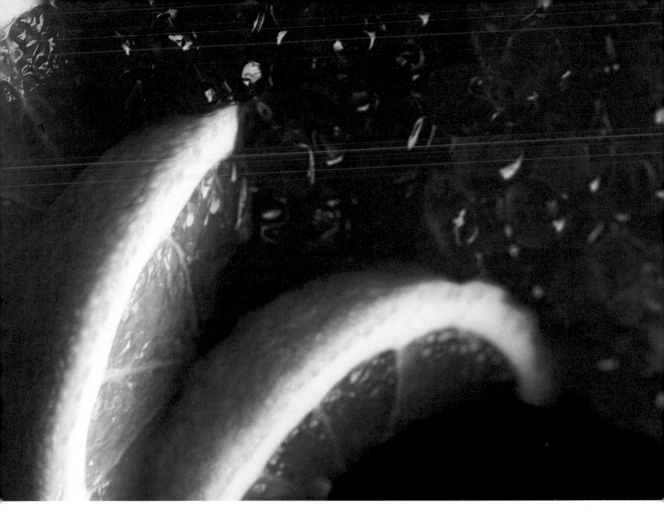

Life at the Peaks

Few women reach their potentials for vitality, clarity, emotional balance and creative power. We're talking about an experience of aliveness where you awaken in the morning feeling great about your life. A state of being that allows you to realize your physical and mental potentials, so your capacity for fun, passion and excitement can soar. Radiant well-being is not just the absence of disease. It is a dynamic state of mind, body and spirit that makes it possible to participate fully and spontaneously in every moment of life.

'What do I think of Western civilisation? I think it would be a very good idea.'

Mahatma Gandhi

STOP THE EPIDEMIC

An epidemic is overtaking the Western world. You need to know about it. Called *insulin resistance syndrome* or *Syndrome X*, it's a serious condition caused primarily by our body's inability to handle the kinds of foods we eat. Syndrome X is not one condition but a collection of abnormalities that tend to occur together. They include high blood pressure, distorted cholesterol parameters and many other medical measurements your doctor worries about: loss of muscle and body tone, an increase in fat, furred arteries, and blood sugar disorders, which produce mood swings. Together, these abnormalities make women vulnerable to overweight and obesity and put us at increased risk of just about every age-related disorder you can name: eye problems, diabetes, heart disease, cancer and Alzheimer's, to mention a few. Syndrome X can be responsible for all sorts of other miseries too – from chronic fatigue and anxiety to irritability, depression and a poor sense of personal worth. Most frightening of all, most women still consider these things to be a 'normal' part of growing older. They are not.

BEWARE SYNDROME X

Syndrome X is not caused by a virus or accident of nature. It's a result of a sedentary lifestyle coupled with the high-grain high-carbohydrate way of eating which we have followed for generations, believing – as government directives still tell us we should – that such a diet constitutes nutrition for health.

Impeccable scientific research indicates that such beliefs are wrong. Eating this way messes up metabolism. Why? Because it is contrary to what, throughout the whole of evolution, your body has been programmed to thrive on, so contrary that it undermines our health and triggers degeneration.

'Symptoms are a way for your body to say, "Listen to me talk for a change."
Carl A. Hammerschlag

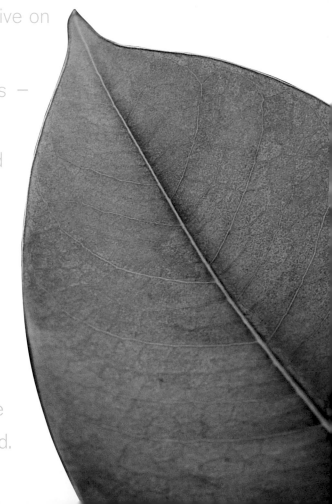

Genes change very slowly. It takes 100,000 years to make even one significant evolutionary change to a gene. The forces of natural selection have acted on us for millions of years, shaping and moulding our genetic make-up and biochemical functioning. As hunter-gatherers, like our predecessors, we have been programmed to thrive on two things:

1 Animal-based protein foods – from eggs and meat to fish.

2 Non-starchy vegetables and herbs, leaves, fruits and seeds (mostly eaten raw).

Our bodies have only been subjected to high-density carbohydrate foods like bread and sugar for the last four thousand years, since agriculture became widespread.

TOO MUCH TOO SOON

Before the agricultural revolution got into full swing, we had never seen flour or bread, starchy vegetables or grains. But with the arrival of the twentieth century we began to flood our systems with these foods. Not long after, convenience foods entered our lives and then took over – foods filled with flour, sugar, junk fats and chemicals. The bottom line is, as a result of our genetic inheritance, some 75 per cent of us just can't handle the onslaught of such 'foreign' fare. It undermines our health and predisposes us to early ageing, obesity and degenerative disease. The widespread incidence of Syndrome X has become a measure of just how destructive a combination of the Western diet plus a sedentary lifestyle has become.

INSULIN STORM

It happens like this: the hormone insulin controls how your body turns carbohydrates into energy. It does this by escorting the glucose in your blood into the cells where it can be turned into ATP (the body's energy currency) within the mitochondria, the cells' energy factories.

Eating too many high-carbohydrate, grain-based and sugar-based foods *floods* your cells with insulin. This leads to a cascade of problems. Your cells lose their sensitivity to insulin. When insulin comes knocking, they don't open to let the glucose in. So your pancreas produces even more insulin. Too much insulin circulating in the blood causes your body to convert glucose into fat, instead of energy, spurring more fat build-up. At the same time, excess insulin prevents your body from releasing stored fat for fuel. It also creates plaque in your arteries, distorts brain chemistry, causing mood swings, and makes your energy unstable.

> '**First the doctor told me the good news: I was going to have a disease named after me...**'
> **Steve Martin**

It's not hard to see that the high-carb diet based on too many grains and sugars (not to mention chemicals the human body does not handle) can lead both directly and indirectly to degeneration, obesity, and the rest of Syndrome X's grim tally.

So much for the bad news. The goods news is actually *magnificent* news. Begin to eat in a way that is as close as possible to what your body has been genetically accustomed to and you can turn your life around. What's more, these foods are absolutely delicious – a far cry from the health-food fodder and the high-carb low-fat stuff that is still too often foisted upon us.

TRANSFORMATIVE TRIAD

An optimal experience of human health and vitality is only possible when what we eat and the way we live is in line with what we have been genetically predisposed to thrive on. Such a simple idea. Yet what dazzling payoffs. It means three things:

● A high-raw diet like that of our hunter-gatherer ancestors.

● Adequate top-quality protein foods.

● A way of eating that is low- or no-grain and low- or no-sugar.

DELICIOUS RADIANCE EATING

At the moment, what is replacing all the high carb stuff in people's minds is high-protein, low-carb eating *à la* Dr Atkins. OK. That's good, or at least it's a step in the right direction. But it does not go far enough. The human body *needs* carbohydrates, but it needs the *right kind* of carbohydrates – carbs friendly to our genes. It also needs *adequate* not *'high'* protein. The carbohydrates we thrive on are found in fresh, raw vegetables, herbs and fresh fruits. Why? Because these are the kinds of carbohydrates our ancestors ate.

THE MISSING PIECES

Twenty years ago we wrote a groundbreaking book about the wonders of high-raw eating called *Raw Energy*. The book quickly became a bestseller. Year after year we are flooded with letters from readers around the world who have discovered the transformative power and payoffs of a high-raw diet.

When we wrote *Raw Energy* we knew nothing about Syndrome X and the fascinating work of Palaeopathologists had yet to be done. Now, thanks to this new scientific information we have been able to add missing pieces to the original *Raw Energy* puzzle. Our understanding of how to combine a high-raw diet with good quality proteins and low-grain eating has resulted in a way of eating that is nothing short of transformational: it slims the body without 'dieting,' strengthens immunity and balances emotions, mind and body. It also helps keep you young, decade after decade.

'Life itself is the proper binge.' **Julia Child**

FACTS YOU SHOULD KNOW

● **Raw Radiance:** Raw foods carry unparalleled power for health and beauty, thanks to the energetic and biochemical order they help create in the body. They carry light energy – photons – gathered by plants and animals from the sun's own energy. These biophotons interact with your body's own light-based, energy-based cellular control and communication systems – your living matrix – to heal, to energize, to bring mental and emotional clarity and to help keep your body strong and resistant to the build-up of toxic waste that invites disease and degeneration.

● **Protein Power:** An all-raw diet is great for short periods as a way of helping the body heal itself. But raw foods are not enough on their own long-term. Yes, people who carry on with an all-raw vegetarian diet for years continue to feel well, but they often lose power and stamina. Many become a bit ungrounded, too. They find it hard to live in the 'real' world. Most people also need enough top-quality protein foods to accompany raw fruits and vegetables. Protein foods, like meat and fish, create the strength for good architecture for body and psyche.

● **Bone Benefits:** New research shows that adequate protein supports healthy bones. Organic and free-range meat, fish, game and eggs contribute enormously to your power and vitality while helping to protect from premature ageing and degenerative disease.

● **Organic Plus:** Today's fruits and vegetables lack yesterday's nutrition. Whenever possible, go for organic foods for better nutrition. They help you avoid toxic build-up from eating foods grown using conventional farming methods, herbicides and pesticides.

'Life is not a problem to be solved, but a mystery to be lived.'
Thomas Merton

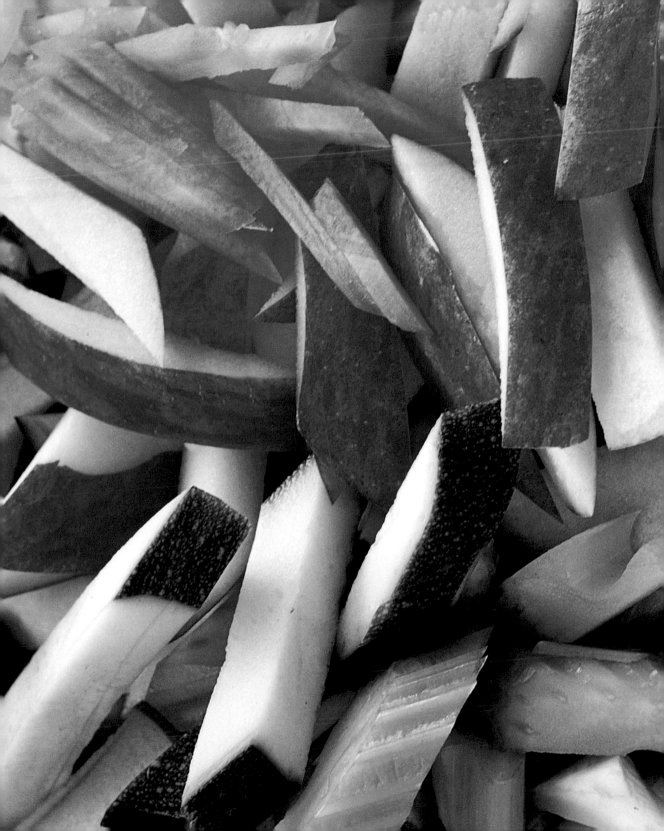

EXPRESS YOUR GENES

Finally – and most important of all – Radiance Eating rebalances metabolism, allowing your body's own remarkable inner power for healing to regenerate and rejuvenate your body and your life. Why? Here it comes again: because a high-raw low-grain diet with adequate protein foods is as close as you can get to eating as our ancestors did.

Radiance Eating, complete with fish, game, herbs and seeds, eggs and meat (preferably organic) or vegan proteins like tofu, makes it possible for the human body to experience élite levels of *genetic expression*. What you may not yet know is that, more important than the genes we have inherited are the ways in which those genes are *expressed*. (This is the scientific term for how your genetic inheritance is lived out day-to-day.) Do your genes express themselves by creating massive vitality? Clarity of mind? Creativity and freedom from illness? Or through chronic fatigue, obesity, sagging skin and spirit, early ageing and degeneration? The quality of your genetic expression depends primarily on how you eat and live, since these determine the quality of the fluids in which your genes bathe within your cells.

NEW LEASE ON LIFE

People who live life at the peaks don't face the future with fears about getting old or falling prey to degenerative disease. They live in anticipation that the best is yet to come. They are no longer ruled by outdated ideas about ageing including illness as a 'natural' part of life. They know different. Their paradigms for ageing are closer to that of world famous age researcher Johan Bjorksten who speaks of giving 'as many people as possible as many more healthy, vigorous years of life as possible'. We call it 'dying young, late in life'.

'I don't feel old – I don't feel anything until noon. Then it's time for my nap.'

Bob Hope

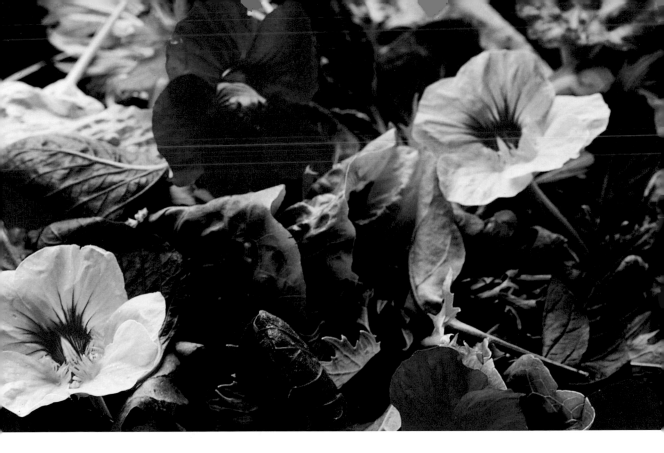

Power and Radiance

Radiance Eating alters the *kind* and *ratio* of the three fundamental nutrients – proteins, carbohydrates and fats – in your diet as well as their *quality*. You eat only the best: slow release, low-density carbohydrates – as many as possible in their raw state – rich in vital plant nutrients and life itself. These foods do not distort blood sugar, upset insulin balance or contribute to Syndrome X. You get plenty of top-quality proteins, omega-3 essential fatty acids and delicious and nutritious oils and fats – from olive oils and flaxseed oil to coconut oil and creamy butter. Its aim is to bring about a *total* and *permanent physical metamorphosis* as well as end fatigue and food cravings. The best news yet? High-raw, low-grain meals are a far cry from what you have come to think of as 'health foods'. You know, the kind of stuff you're 'supposed' to eat even though it tastes revolting. These foods are real foods – absolutely delicious – splendid herb salads with shavings of the best Parmesan, fish or chicken cooked in a rich coconut sauce, even natural desserts and treats if you have a sweet tooth. Eat them and enjoy, while your body gets busy making itself healthier, more radiant and more beautiful with each week that passes.

7 EAT RADIANCE
simple...irresistible...life-changing

Become a radiance eater. Whether you choose to ease gracefully into this new food style or jump right in, here you'll find all the information you need to transform your life with the highest level of biochemical and energetic order. Get into the foods your cells crave. Then graze to your heart's content as you break through to a new dimension of well-being.

Serious about living your life at the peaks? The first job of the day is to empty your cupboards, fridge and freezer of energy-depleting foods. These include biscuits and pasta, breakfast cereals, jams and preserves, convenience foods, ice-cream, packaged fruit drinks and frozen convenience meals. Get rid of anything which might tempt you to fall back into old habits.

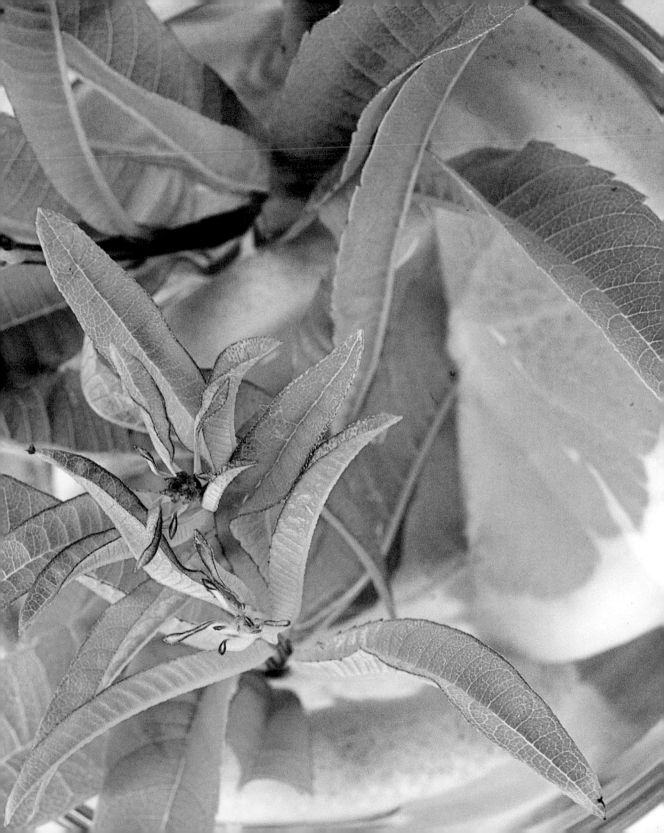

FORAGE AT THE EDGE

Next, stock up on radiance fodder. The most important foods for vitality and good looks are these: fresh, non-starchy vegetables, fruits and proteins like meat, seafood, eggs and game, as well as micro-filtered whey (see Resources), maybe a little unprocessed cheese and soy proteins, like tofu, if you're vegetarian. You'll find most of the healthiest, freshest, and most natural foods around the outside edges of your supermarket or organic emporium. The ready-in-a-minute, pre-made stuff hovers in the inner isles. Natural, wholesome foods tend towards the outside as they are perishable and therefore have to be replaced often. Choose a wide variety of vegetables and fruits and plan to eat most of them raw.

10 TIPS FOR RADIANCE EATING

Choose your foods for two reasons: because they are irresistibly delicious and because they can supply you with the highest possible support biochemically and energetically for beauty and health.

● Steer clear of grain-based carbohydrate foods for one month while your body is adjusting to Radiance Eating. These include flour, breakfast cereals, pasta, breads, and all forms of sugar. Afterwards, if you like, add back *whole* grains bit by bit in the form of brown rice, porridge made from jumbo oats, buckwheat noodles and whole grain bread (preferably made from 100% rye, oats or spelt, instead of wheat or maize).

● Eat plenty of natural, fresh, organic vegetables and fruits. Non-starchy vegetables high in phytonutrients and antioxidants are your primary source of carbohydrates.

● Enjoy one or two large radiant salads a day – glorious combinations of fresh herbs, green leaves, crunchy peppers, sprouts, carrots, apples and anything else splendid and delicious you can lay your hands on, plus good-quality protein foods like chicken, fish or organic eggs or tofu.

● Cut out soft drinks, packaged fruit juices, all processed drinks and alcohol, except for an occasional glass or two of good wine.

● Use cold-pressed extra-virgin olive oil, walnut oil, and flaxseed oil on your salads, and butter, coconut oil (great for skin) or olive oil for cooking.

● Eat oily fish three times a week. It contains the omega-3 fatty acids DHA and EPA to keep skin glowing and protect your body from early ageing.

● Steer clear of margarine, processed and highly hydrogenated vegetable oils and any sauces or salad dressings that contain them. They can screw up hormones and undermine health.

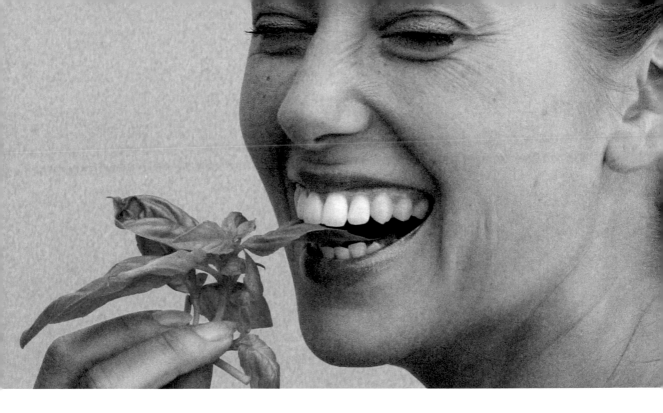

● Eat good-quality proteins like fresh fish, free-range chicken, eggs, game, organic meat, tofu and micro-filtered whey twice a day.

● Coffee? Limit yourself to one cup a day.

● Eliminate sweeteners, including sugar, malt extract, corn syrup, and chemical sweeteners. Limit your use of honey to a teaspoonful or two a day (Manuka honey is best).

BREAKTHROUGH

Want to find out fast how transforming radiance eating is and just how much it can do for you? For the first month completely cut out all grain-based foods. This gives your body the opportunity to rebalance insulin and blood sugar, and clear fatigue and cravings as quickly as possible. Afterwards, if you feel you need or want some grain foods (about 20 per cent of women do) then add small amounts of only the best grains and flours. You can also add in the odd potato or sweet potato, but as these quickly turn into a lot of glucose in the blood they are best kept for special treats. Last word: go for a 30-minute walk each day. This too helps restore good insulin sensitivity, stabilizes blood sugar and clears signs of Syndrome X.

'It is now proved beyond a doubt that ageing is one of the leading causes of statistics.'

Unknown

SWEETENERS

The best sweetener in the world comes from a South American plant called Stevia. Sadly it is no longer available in the EU for regulatory reasons to do with the lobbying power of chemical companies that sell artificial sweeteners. Artificial sweeteners are chemicals foreign to your body and potentially dangerous. Do not use them or eat or drink anything that contains them. Many studies show that they can have a dangerous effect on living organisms when used regularly. If you can get Stevia, use it. It is 300 times sweeter than sugar itself and *good* for you. It comes in many varieties, the best is the organic Stevita Spoonable Stevia which you use just as you would use ordinary sugar, although you will need far less of it (see Resources).

Manuka honey is another alternative for sweetening. It has far greater molecular density than any other form of honey. This makes it behave differently in the body in relation to the insulin/glucose axis. Used in moderate amounts it does not have the same insulin unbalancing effect that other honeys, sugars, malt extracts and the rest do. It also has remarkable anti-bacterial and anti-viral properties.

IT TASTES BEST – BUY IT

Whenever possible, go organic. Not only do organic fruits, vegetables and protein goods taste better, the organic matter in healthy soil is nature's factory for biological activity and biophoton order. Organic foods bring you the best balance of minerals, trace elements, vitamins and phytonutrients. They also make plants grown on them highly resistant to disease – a benefit they pass on to you when you eat them.

RAW TRUTHS

Aim to eat at least 50 per cent of your foods in their natural raw state. When you are under stress increase that percentage to 75 per cent. From sashimi to strawberries, clean, wholesome foods eaten raw have remarkable health-enhancing and anti-ageing properties. This is why they are used for healing and rejuvenation at the most famous natural clinics and spas around the world. Uncooked foods improve micro-circulation, cellular functioning and DNA expression. Making a high percentage of what you eat raw heightens your energy and stamina, supplies a high level of bio-photon order to the living matrix, counters ageing and brings you the best natural antioxidant support you can get anywhere.

Natural food emporiums are great places to find good organic vegetables and other produce, as well as eggs, meat, dairy products and fish, from animals that have not been stuffed full of antibiotics, dipped in chemicals or treated with hormones. Try to shop as much as possible in stores that offer organic produce and untreated food.

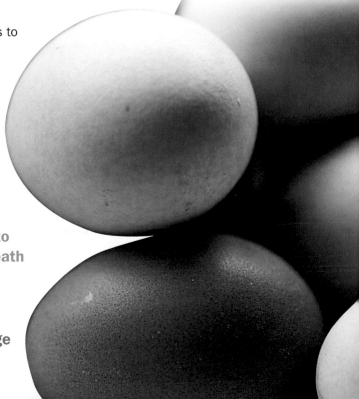

'I remember when people used to step outside a moment for a breath of fresh air. Now sometimes you have to step outside for days before you get it.'

Victor Borge

GREAT CHOICES – FRESH STUFF

Full of biophoton order, phytonutrient power and fibre, these fresh living fruits and vegetables are also just plain delicious.

Salad Stuff Raw/ Cooked	Vegetables Cooked	Fresh Fruit
Alfalfa sprouts	Artichoke	Apple
Avocados	Asparagus	Apricots
Bamboo shoots	Aubergine	Blueberries
Bell peppers	Beans (green)	Boysenberries
Broccoli	Bok choy	Cantaloupe melon
Cabbage	Broccoli	Cherries
Capsicum	Brussels sprouts	Grapefruit
Cauliflower	Cabbage	Honeydew melon
Celery	Cauliflower	Kiwi fruit
Cucumber	Chick peas	Lemon
Endive	Collard greens	Lime
Escarole	Courgette	Mandarin
Fennel	Kale	Nectarine
Lettuce	Leeks	Orange
Mushrooms	Lentils	Peach
Onions	Mushrooms	Pear
Radishes	Okra	Plum
Rocket	Onions	Pineapple
Salsa	Sauerkraut	Raspberries
Snow peas	Silver beet	Strawberries
Spinach	Spinach	Tangerine
Sprouted seeds	Turnip	Watermelon
String beans	Yellow squash	
Tomato		

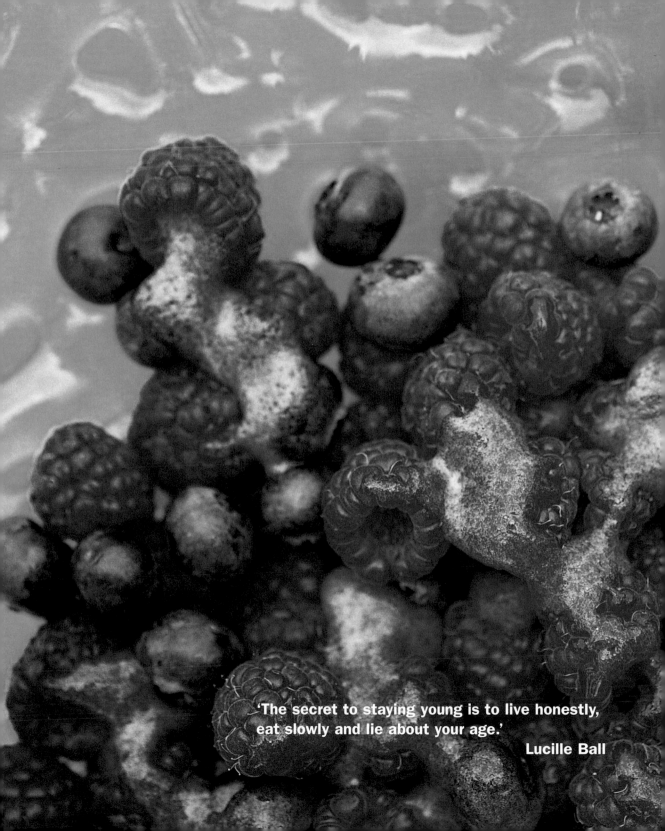

'The secret to staying young is to live honestly, eat slowly and lie about your age.'

Lucille Ball

Power Proteins

Radiance Eating calls for a few more protein foods than you may have been used to. This is important. The single most widespread deficiency of macronutrients as people get older comes from eating too little good-quality protein. Scientists once believed that we had to be careful not to eat too much protein. Any excess, it was thought, would leach calcium from bones and make us prone to osteoporosis. Several large-scale studies have now proved this idea wrong. In fact it is a *lack* of sufficient protein that predisposes us to bone thinning. As women get older they often eat less meat, fish, eggs and other protein foods. Yet these are exactly the kind of foods we need to support our immune system and keep our hormone levels from flagging, not to mention to enhance lean body mass and keep skin firm and youthful.

STRENGTH FOODS

GOOD CHOICE PROTEINS (ALL ORGANIC)	POOR CHOICE PROTEINS
Meat and Poultry	
Beef, lean	Bacon
Beef, minced (less than 15% fat)	Beef, fatty cuts
Chicken breast	
Lamb	Pepperoni
Lamb's liver	Salami
Turkey breast	Sausage: pork, beef, turkey or chicken
Fish and Seafood	
(Buy fish that is as fresh as possible and is from sustainable sources)	Processed fish such as:
Bass	Breaded fish
Bluefish Calamari	Crab cakes
Clams	Surimi
Cod *	
Crab	There's no harm in having the odd
Grouper	slice of naturally smoked salmon. But
Haddock	the more food is processed, the less
Halibut	it supports high-level health.
Lobster	

Mackerel *
Prawns
Salmon *
Sardines *
Scallops
Snapper
Squid
Swordfish
Trout *
Tuna, canned in water
Tuna, steak *
* = good sources of omega-3 fats.

Eggs

If possible, buy organic, if not, at least free-range. Eat them any way you like: soft and hard-boiled, in omelettes, poached, scrambled or fried. Don't worry about the cholesterol scares from eggs. They have been proved to be unfounded.

Cheese (Eat occasionally)

Parmesan
Camembert
Feta
Cottage cheese, low fat
Ricotta
Mozzarella

Note: stay away from any and all processed cheeses.

Micro-filtered Whey

The finest protein in the world. It comes in powdered form and is great for smoothies. Good for vegetarians and non-vegetarians alike (see Resources).

Vegan Options

Tofu
Tempeh
Miso
Soy milk and other soy products

Omega-3 Fats for Beauty

Try to eat oily fish at least three times a week. Their omega-3 fatty acids, DHA and EPA, are fantastic for beautiful skin and healthy joints. Your body can absorb the omega-3s in wild salmon, mackerel, sardines, tuna and herrings directly. Omega-3s help balance hormones, protect from degeneration, and have powerful anti-inflammatory properties. Flaxseed oil is also a good source of omega-3 fatty acids. But it differs from fish oil. Flaxseed contains a lot of linolenic acid, which is the precursor to DHA and EPA. The problem is, some people can't convert linolenic acid into useable DHA and EPA and for them, the omega-3s from fish are a better choice. Make sure you eat plenty of both oily fish and flaxseed oil.

GOOD-GUY FATS

These are the healthiest available. Use them for cooking, in salad dressings and for snacks. Include about a tablespoon or so in each meal from the list below. In addition to the fat you get from food, use two teaspoons of flaxseed oil every day on your salads and consider taking a good omega-3 EPA and DHA fish oils supplement. A word of warning: you can pour flaxseed oil on cooked vegetables, yoghurt, or use it in salads, but never use it for cooking as heat destroys its value.

- extra-virgin olive oil
- coconut oil
- butter
- avocados (and guacamole)
- almonds and almond butter
- macadamia nuts and macadamia butter
- olives
- tahini

When choosing dairy food, remember that butter, although not a source of essential fatty acids, is perfectly respectable – far better than margarine. In general go for low-fat dairy products – cottage cheese, ricotta, mascarpone, and unsweetened yoghurt. Eat cream or soured cream as a special treat now and then. Stay away from flavoured cottage cheeses, yoghurts and other dairy products which are usually loaded with sugar or other sweeteners, as well as questionable flavourings.

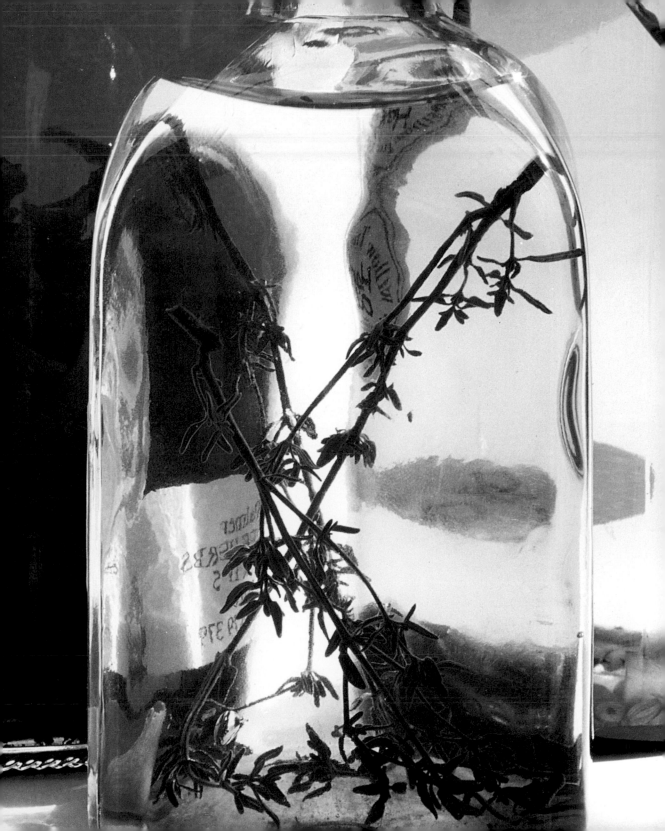

POOR-CHOICE CARBOHYDRATES

Here are the foods to avoid during your first month on Radiance Eating. After that, have them only occasionally.

Vegetables Cooked	Grains, Cereals, Bread	Condiments and Treats
Baked beans	Bagels	Barbecue sauce
Chips (potato)	Biscuits	Cocktail sauce
Lima beans	Breadcrumbs	Ice-cream
Pinto beans	Bread sticks	Jam or jelly
Potatoes	Bread , wholegrain or white	Relish, pickle
Refried beans	Bulgar wheat	Sugar in all forms
Sweet potatoes	Cereal	Sweets
	Cornflour	Syrups
	Couscous	Teriyaki sauce
	Crackers	Tomato sauce
	Croissants	
	Croutons	
	Doughnuts	
	Granola	
	Melba toast	
	Millet	
	Muffins/cakes	

'Tomorrow is a new day; begin it well and serenely and with too high a spirit to be encumbered with your old nonsense.'

Ralph Waldo Emerson

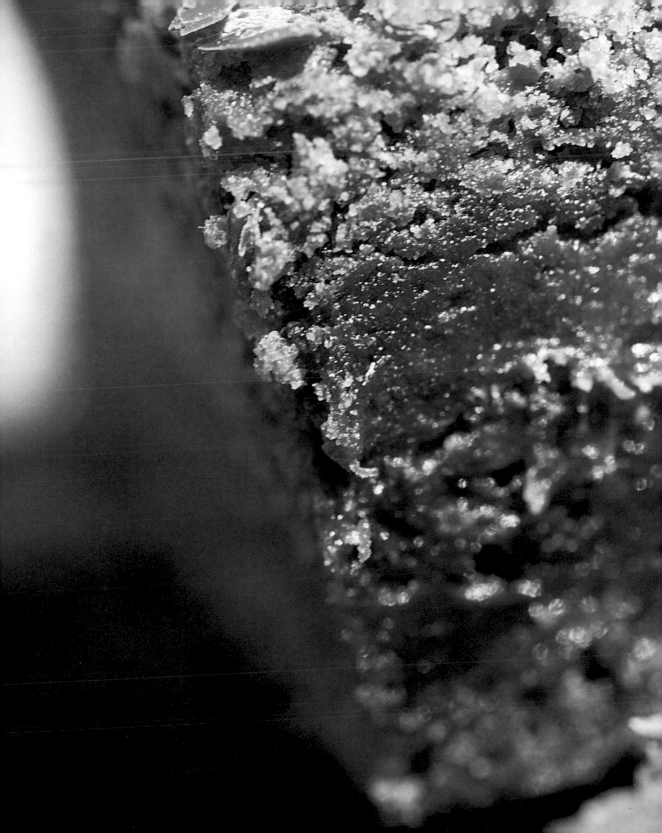

Eating for Radiance

Radiance Eating starts here. There is no need to stick rigidly to a menu plan or count calories, carbs, fats and proteins to reap the benefits. Within a couple of weeks your energy begins to rise. After another two weeks, as your body detoxes and readjusts, you begin to sense intuitively which foods work best for you and which don't. Listen to those internal messages. If your appetite has been excessive, you'll find it normalizes naturally as the nutrient-rich foods you are eating nourish you better than ever before.

Just follow the principles outlined above and check out the meal suggestions below. The best ways to cook your food are to grill, steam, bake, wok-fry or sauté. See how you get on with red meat. Some women, especially as they get older, find they don't handle it well but do better with fish. Others find they thrive on red meat even though most of their lives they may have avoided it because they were told it was bad for them. Experiment to discover what works for you.

salad mastery

If you find yourself reluctantly reaching for microwave dinners because you 'don't have time for a healthy meal', master the art of *authentic fast food*. You can prepare a mouth-watering whole-meal, protein-rich salad that leaves you satisfied and feeling great in 10 minutes or less. Here's how:

Shop for Beauty

Great salads start in the shopping stage. Buy what's most beautiful – as much as possible organic. Forget the rest. When you get your vegetables home, wash and dry them thoroughly. Then store them in large, clear, air-tight plastic bags or bins in the fridge. We like to add a couple of drops of cold water to each bag/bin, which can help keep even lettuces and herbs fresh for a whole week.

Once your vegetables are ready to go, salad-making happens almost instantly. Simply pull out two, three or four bins full of lovely bright-coloured fresh foods and dive in.

Protein Choice

Begin each whole-meal salad by deciding which protein you'll use. Fresh salmon? Tinned tuna? Chicken breast? Prawns? Diced hard-boiled egg? Put your protein food on to cook (if necessary) while you prepare your vegetables. We keep fish, chicken breasts and baby squid for salads frozen in the freezer and cook them up in a little olive oil or coconut oil while we chop the other ingredients. Whenever you cook meat, poultry or fish, make sure there's enough for leftovers to make light work of your salad preparation the next day.

Salad-making

Make your salad from a variety of vegetables and textures – finely shredded red cabbage, with julienned celeriac and coarsely grated apple, for instance. Or finely chopped spinach with chunks of avocado, chopped tomatoes and sliced radishes. We often eat vegetables most people would cook, like broccoli and cauliflower, raw in salads. Or we may blanch broccoli/cauliflower florets for a few seconds in a bowl of boiling water to bring out their flavour, then add them to raw vegetables. In the wintertime especially, when good organic vegetables are hard to come by, we grow our own sprouted seeds from marrowfat peas, chickpeas, lentils, broccoli and radish seeds. They are packed with nutrients, tasty, inexpensive and have a great fridge shelf life. You can often buy them ready-sprouted from your health food emporium.

Lazy Dressing

Making salad dressing can be time-consuming. Instead, we use an Italian trick and simply dress the salad directly in the bowl: a few tablespoons of extra-virgin olive oil, some chopped fresh herbs, crushed raw garlic, a dash of Worcestershire sauce, some Maldon salt or a dash of tamari, the juice of a lemon or a couple of tablespoons of wine vinegar or balsamic vinegar, some Cajun seasoning and freshly ground course black pepper. We might also add salad sprinkles, such as cashews, hazelnuts, pumpkin seeds, sesame seeds, sunflower seeds, feta cheese or Parmesan.

Top and Go

When your protein choice is ready, top your salad with it and enjoy! Once you get into the swing of Salad Mastery you'll love how fun, simple and delicious eating this way is.

MANDOLIN MAGIC

The one piece of kitchen equipment we would never be without is a mandolin. The best have a V-shaped blade, into which fit plastic inserts, with various 'knives' (see Resources). You can julienne, make chip-size chunks, slice thin or thick. Unlike conventional graters, which tend to mash vegetables and fruits, a mandolin slices them cleanly. It's important to use the hand protector device, which comes with every model. (We both know this from bloody experience!)

RADIANCE MEAL SUGGESTIONS

Let's look at a few suggestions for breakfast, lunch, dinner and snacks. The menus that follow are only meant to get you started. They'll give you a feel for radiance eating. If you want to change your eating habits gradually, start by adding a radiance meal to your normal diet every day or two. If, like us, you like to jump into things feet first, spend a day or two cleaning out your cupboards. Refill your fridge with radiance foods. Then launch into it with unbridled passion. Balance things so you get good-quality proteins, fats, and fresh raw vegetables or fruit at every meal. You will be delighted with the changes you experience.

Breakfasts:

● **Omelette with Fresh Vegetables:** Cook your omelette in butter or olive oil and toss in chopped tomatoes, peppers and spinach. Serve with a slice of cantaloupe melon or honeydew.

● **Very Berry Frappé:** Blend 20 to 30 grams of micro-filtered whey protein powder, a teaspoon of flaxseed oil, chopped apple, chopped pear or a handful of berries, soy milk or water plus a few ice cubes. It can have you out of the door in a New York minute.

● **Grilled Fish:** Salmon is especially good with garlic and sweet onions. Enjoy with a bowl of mixed berries, some melon or an apple.

● **Unsweetened Yoghurt:** Combine regular or soy yoghurt with fresh fruit and sprinkle with slivered almonds.

● **Real Bircher Muesli:** Soak overnight 2 to 3 tablespoons of jumbo porridge oats or raw buckwheat in water. Next morning add 1 teaspoon to 1 dessertspoon of coconut oil, an apple or pear (chopped or grated) and a handful of fresh or frozen berries. Sweeten with Manuka honey or stevia if desired.

● **Old-fashioned Porridge:** Cook jumbo oats in water and salt to taste. Top with a grated apple, banana or fresh or frozen blueberries. Sprinkle with cinnamon and add a dab of butter if you like.

● **Vanilla Nog:** Blend soy milk with a handful of raw cashews, half a teaspoon of vanilla extract, 1 teaspoon ground cinnamon, – 1/2 teaspoon nutmeg, and one banana for a rich and creamy smoothie.

'During one of our trips through Afghanistan, we lost our corkscrew. We had to live on food and water for several days.'
W.C. Fields

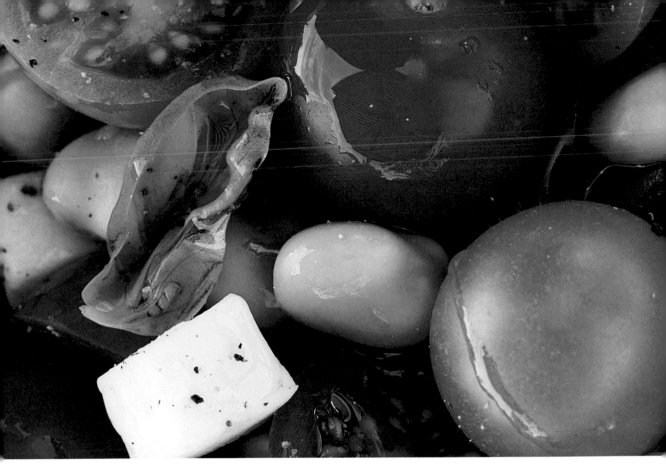

Lunches:

- **Chicken or Turkey Spinach Salad:** Combine slices of chicken or turkey breast with diced yellow, red and green peppers, sweet red onions and sliced fresh mushrooms. Top with grated hard-boiled eggs. Toss with olive oil, lemon and Dijon mustard dressing.

- **Souvlaki Kebabs:** Skewer lamb or chicken chunks with onion pieces and crunchy vegetables, dip in olive oil and season with herbs and fresh lemon juice, then grill. Serve on a bed of shredded raw greens.

- **Radiance Crudités:** Enjoy sticks of carrots, celery, cucumber and other raw vegetables dipped in a selection of guacamole, hummus and aubergine dips.

- **Fresh Grilled Tuna:** Serve tuna on a bed of rocket, with black olives and herbs. Enjoy with a mixed salad dressed with olive oil, balsamic vinegar and garlic dressing.

- **Greek Feta Salad:** Combine left-over chicken or lamb with lettuce, cucumber and diced tomato. Sprinkle with sunflower seeds, pumpkin seeds, Greek olives and crumbled feta cheese. Dress with olive oil, lemon and fresh garlic.

- **Fruit and Protein Plate:** Fill cos lettuce leaves with low-fat cottage cheese and serve with slices of fresh peaches, apricots, oranges and French dressing.

Dinners:

● **Sautéed Sea Bass:** Serve with steamed broccoli and courgettes with slivered almonds, herb salad, sliced oranges and shaved coconut. Try strawberries with fresh lemon juice and mint for dessert.

● **Turkey Burger:** Combine minced turkey with finely chopped green onions or scallions and red pepper. Grill with courgettes, onion slices and a Portobello mushroom or two. Serve with slivered raw beetroot and apple salad dressed with orange juice and curry powder.

● **Grilled Organic Beef Patty:** Pat into shape, season with fresh ground pepper and capers and grill. Serve with green beans and spinach spiked with lemon juice, plus crudités - cucumbers, tomatoes, celery, and crunchy lettuce with salsa dip.

● **Prawn Rocket Salad:** Toss rocket leaves with grilled prawns and Greek olives. Dress with olive oil, lemon juice and garlic and top with slivers of Parmesan. Enjoy with fresh blackberries and raspberries for dessert.

● **Stir-Fried Chicken:** Wok-fry chicken with bok choy, bean sprouts, ginger, green onions, garlic and water chestnuts in coconut oil. Add a coconut cream sauce and sprinkle with toasted sesame seeds. Serve with a red cabbage coleslaw with onions, garlic and apple. Enjoy with melon balls and fresh ginger for dessert.

Snacks:

Judge for yourself whether or not snacks work for you. For some people they are terrific, for others eating more often than every 4 to 5 hours increases insulin resistance and leads to food cravings. Play it by ear. Here are some suggestions for good quality snacks:

- ● Half a chicken breast
- ● An apple, an orange, a pear or a few strawberries
- ● A handful of raw, unsalted cashews, almonds, brazils, hazelnuts, sunflower seeds, walnuts, macadamia nuts
- ● A few crudités splashed with lemon, soy sauce and a bit of olive oil
- ● 1 ounce of sunflower seeds, walnuts, macadamias, almonds
- ● A hard-boiled egg
- ● A smoothie made with 10 to 15 grams of protein from micro-filtered whey
- ● A cup of low-fat cottage cheese

NUTRITIONAL SUPPLEMENTS

We recommend the following daily:

● A good multiple vitamin including phytonutrients and B Complex (see Resources). 1000 – 3000mg omega-3 EPA and DHA fish oils in capsule form (see Resources) if you eat fatty fish less than once a day.

● 100 – 200mg Alpha Lipoic Acid.

ALA supports the age-reversing powers of Radiance Eating. It is 400 times stronger than vitamins C and E and raises the levels of these two vitamins in your body. It also counters inflammatory reactions. ALA:

● Protects from premature ageing.
● Improves insulin sensitivity.
● Enhances immunity.
● Reduces the cross-linking of collagen.
● Neutralizes free radicals.

New Life Starts Here

Radiance Eating leads to a whole new way of being. You become more alert and more active. You may sleep less, yet better, as your system becomes clearer of toxicity. You find yourself better able to deal with stress. High-raw, low-grain eating provides you with optimal levels of potassium, rapidly restoring your body's important sodium-potassium balance. This increases resistance to fatigue and brings a greater feeling of calm and stability. Radiance Eating may set you slightly apart from your gravy-eating, hard-drinking friends. It may even have them feeling slightly suspicious of you in the beginning. But as soon as they find you are not trying to sell them anything – thanks of course to your live-and-let-live attitude – they will not only show respect for your new lifestyle, the people around you who were once the most resistant and the most opinionated can be the first to become intrigued by what Radiance Eating has to offer. And thanks to their strong independent streak, they are often the ones with the energy, interest and determination to try it for themselves.

8 POWERSLIM
get lean for life

Radiance Eating makes weight control easy. High-raw, low-grain eating banishes cravings and helps clear addictions. It also paves the way to feeling really good about yourself and your body. Ordinary weight-loss diets are notoriously unsuccessful long-term. Going on and off them creates sub-clinical deficiencies leading to fatigue and 'hidden hunger'. Slimming foods, including low-calorie, grain-based fare and processed, packaged meals, disturb insulin balance, create food addictions, cause binge eating and lead to even more weight gain down the road. One of the blessings of Radiance Eating is that you never end up looking drawn and flabby as you shed excess fat naturally. Skin and muscles get firm. Your whole body undergoes a process of rejuvenation.

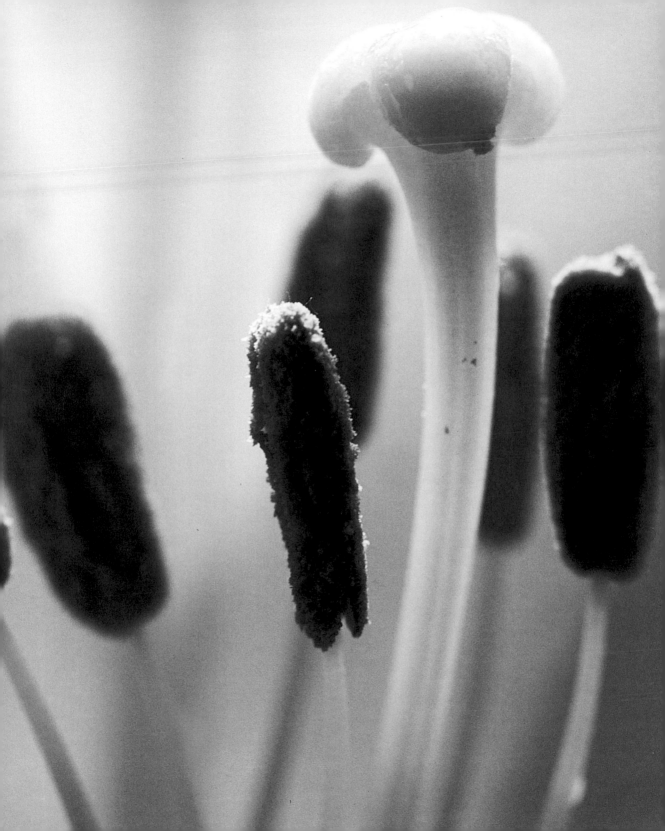

'I went on a diet, swore off drinking and heavy eating, and in fourteen days I had lost exactly two weeks.'

Joe E. Lewis

In the so-called civilized world, people are fatter than ever. What's worse, we grow fatter still with each year that passes. Food manufacturers, government bodies and well-meaning doctors urge us to eat more low-fat high-carb foods: bread and cereals, rice and pasta. Fats, not carbohydrates, are supposed to be the villains that make us fat. Only they're *not.* Extensive research into the effects of a low-fat, high-carb diet on insulin resistance, obesity and the development of degenerative diseases, shows conclusively that these are precisely the foods that make us fat in the first place.

The more industrialized and commercial our societies have become, the more processed foods we eat and the more our blood sugar and insulin levels soar. It is because of this effect that these foods become highly addictive. Eat one biscuit and you can end up wanting to devour the whole packet. Carbohydrate craving is the name of the game – the constant or intermittent hunger that people on a high-carb diet suffer. Such behaviour is not the consequence of a lack of willpower, but the result of imbalances in the body – especially in insulin and blood sugar – caused by a diet too high in sugar, flour and foods made from them.

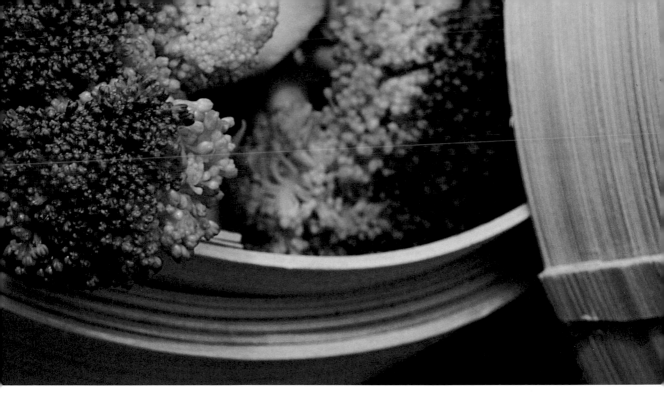

THE RIGHT CARBS

The more cooked and processed, carbohydrate-dense, sugar-creating foods you eat, the more insulin you produce. The more insulin you produce, the more weight you tend to gain – that is if, like the majority of people, you have inherited a genetic tendency to store energy as fat in your body. By contrast, low-density carbs – vegetables like broccoli, spinach and Chinese leaves – have 4 to 10 times less blood sugar-unbalancing carbohydrate than pastas, breakfast cereals and breads. You can eat huge quantities of low-carbohydrate-dense foods without having to wrestle with insulin-related health problems.

There's another weight-gain issue too. Eating too many nutritionally 'empty' convenience foods and too few nutritionally supportive ones, overloads your digestive system. This in turn leads to enzyme deficiencies so you can't break down foods fully to provide nutrients for your cells to use. Then, no matter how much you eat, you feel plagued by constant hunger, since your body is not able to assimilate the nutrients it needs from the foods you eat to enable it to thrive.

RADIANCE LEAN

The high-raw, low-grain approach to weight loss works *with* nature rather than against it. It brings superb nutrition and allows you to lose unwanted pounds slowly and steadily. You don't need to count calories, buy packaged 'slimming meals', or weigh out bird-sized portions on kitchen scales. You will feel neither deprived nor guilty when you eat. Strength, clarity of mind, confidence and a sense of well-being that makes you want to do what is best for your body are just some of the rewards.

NO MORE CRAVINGS

Radiance Eating means you need never go hungry nor feel deprived. Women who try it report that their cravings for sugary and high-carb foods completely disappear after a few days. This is because your body acts quickly to stabilize blood sugar levels. As it does, you tap into higher levels of energy. Your skin loses its puffiness by releasing excess water in the tissues as part of the detoxification process. And – joy of joys – addictive eating completely disappears in most people. But hear this: it takes three to five days of Radiance Eating for your body to adjust and for this to happen. During the first few days you may find your cravings continue. If so, eat more protein foods as snacks and at meal times. Rest a bit more while your body is making the changeover. And be assured: freedom from cravings is on its way.

VICIOUS CYCLE

To digest foods we rely on enzymes – plenty of them – of just the right kind. Eating the wrong food, or eating too much, depletes your body and stresses the whole system. This can result in food allergies and sub-clinical vitamin and mineral deficiencies, which in turn reinforce the vicious cycle of hidden hunger. Radiance Eating clears most of these problems. It is fabulous for weight loss for another reason too. It powerfully protects against Syndrome X, correcting insulin balance so your body does not lay down fat stores. Drinking lots of water (see p.116) is an essential part of shedding fat from your body as well. It enhances enzyme functions, detoxifies and even calms hunger.

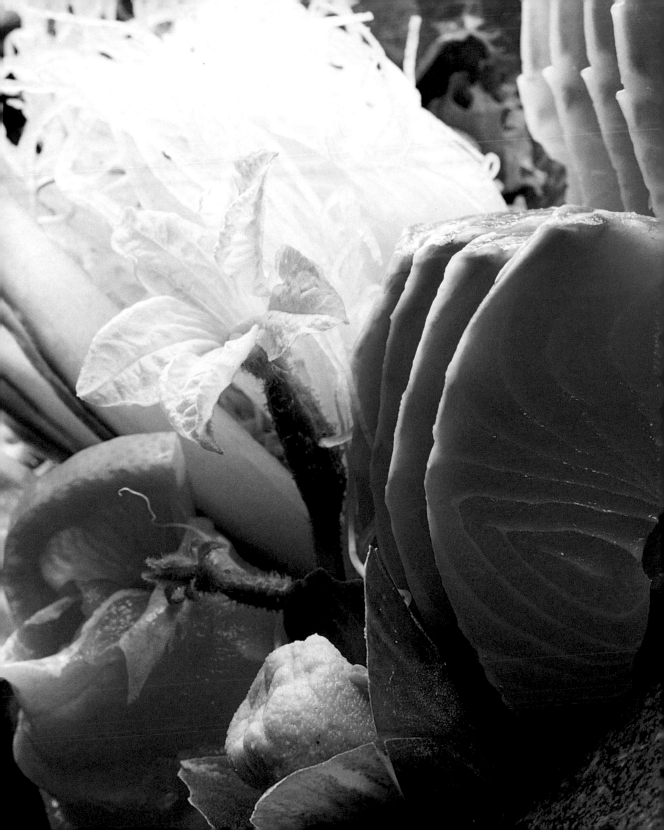

Hunger Can Be Thirst

The control centre for both thirst and hunger is in the same place in your body: the hypothalamus. Often when you think you are hungry what your body is trying to tell you is that you need to take in more water. Perhaps the best-kept secret in the world about weight control is this: reach for a glass of water every time you feel hungry between meals and you will find your hunger diminishing within minutes. Try it and see.

There is another way in which drinking optimal quantities of water plays a central role in fat loss. It has to do with your kidneys. The kidneys are responsible for recycling all the water in your body – some 800 glasses of it a day – and for filtering out any wastes before they can lower immunity, create fatigue, or make you feel hungry (even though you have had enough to eat) and cause the kind of water retention that plagues serial dieters. The filtering mechanism responsible for all this in the kidneys is made up of millions of microscopic bodies known as glomeruli. They identify waste products like urea as well as screening out other chemicals and unwanted metals and minerals. At the same time they pour back into the bloodstream the minerals you do need and regulate your body's acid-alkaline balance.

DRINK LIKE A FISH

When some part of you needs more water, it's your kidneys' job to make sure it arrives. For instance, when you are hot and sweating a message is sent to the pituitary gland telling it to release the anti-diuretic hormone which in turn tells your kidneys to let more water be reabsorbed into the blood. At such times, your urine can become highly concentrated and dark in colour. But provided you replenish the water you are losing in sweat by drinking more, your kidneys remain happy and well-functioning and the appetite/thirst messages from your brain do not become confused. When your body's water level gets too low from not drinking enough, your kidneys cannot carry out their cleansing efficiently. Then your liver has to come to the rescue, trying not to let the side down. The trouble is the liver's main function in weight loss is to mobilize body fat and help transform it into usable energy. When it has to take on some of the kidneys' work the liver is unable to do its fat-mobilizing job effectively. Drinking lots of water – far more than you think you need – helps your kidneys to help your liver to help you lose weight.

'Do I look heavyish to you? I feel heavyish. Put a note on my desk in the morning, "Think thin"'.

Cary Grant to his secretary, *North by Northwest*

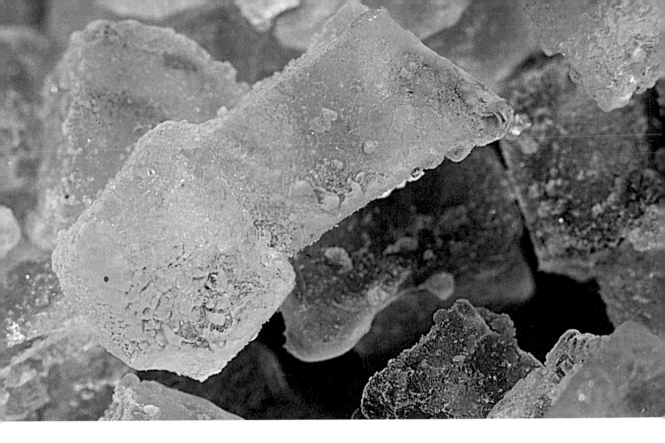

BANISH SUGAR AND CARB CRAVINGS

The non-essential amino acid L-glutamine can be a great help while your insulin and blood sugar are rebalancing, if you are temporarily bothered by a desire to eat sweets or grain-based carb foods. It is a white, largely tasteless powder that in addition to banishing cravings has all sorts of other great effects. It:

- reduces fatigue
- improves endurance when you exercise
- benefits the liver and intestines
- strengthens the immune system
- enhances mental functions

Take it on an *empty stomach*. Mix into a glass of water or just put the powder on your tongue and use the water as a chaser. Usual dose is 1 gramme at a time to calm cravings.

Fat Is Dead

Animal bodies, like ours, are made up of two basic components – *lean body mass* (LBM), which encompasses our muscle tissue, and *fat*. Lean body mass consists of organs like the heart, the liver, the pancreas, bones and skin, as well as muscle. It is your LBM that burns oxygen, uses nutrients from your food, thinks and feels, moves, grows and repairs itself. A high percentage of LBM is what gives wild animals their power, ease of movement, stamina and sleek bodies. The rest of you is fat.

Your body's fat stores are metabolically *inactive*. They don't burn calories. Only mitochondria – the energy factories in your muscle cells – do this. The reason your body stores fat at all is to provide it with reserves of potential energy through the lean times when food is not available. People who have inherited what is known as the *thrifty gene* have a genetic tendency to store fat. Their ancestors were the ones that lasted through those long cold winters when everyone else was dying of starvation. This thrifty gene is not of great benefit to those of us now in developed countries who don't face starvation. Storing excess fat makes us highly prone to degenerative conditions including obesity, diabetes and overall body wastage and weakness known as *sarcopenia*.

> 'Never eat at a single sitting more than you can lift.'
>
> **Miss Piggy**

MUSCLE FOR TRANSFORMATION

Your LBM is always changing – increasing or decreasing. When it changes this is not because of alterations in your organs or bones but rather because of alterations in your muscle. Under-muscled people have low levels of energy. Studies show they are at as great a risk from degeneration and early ageing as people who are over-fat. When muscles are in tone, your posture is good too, for posture depends on muscle alone. So does the proper elimination of waste from your cells. The lymphatic system which carries waste products away is not powered by the heart but by muscle movement. The more muscle movement you get the better it works. This is particularly important for women – even slim women. For unless your lymphatic system is working properly you can end up with deposits of water, wastes and fat on localized areas of your body, better known as cellulite.

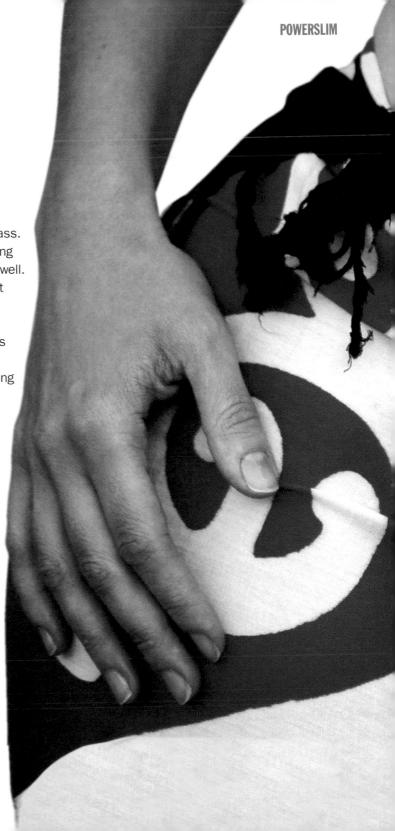

USE IT OR LOSE IT

Yo-yo dieting destroys lean body mass. You lose weight, but instead of losing only fat you lose muscle tissue as well. When the inevitable rebound weight gain takes place, you don't regain muscle tissue, only fat. Radiance Eating is not about weight loss. It is about permanent *fat* loss. It decreases fat stores while enhancing muscle. Break your arm and it will shed half of its muscle and a third of its bone mass within a few weeks, simply because you stop using it. If you are forced for any reason to stay in bed for a few months, the loss of minerals from your bones and ageing of your muscle tissue can speed up by ten years. That is the bad news. The good news is that your body responds amazingly to exercise, even to a little of it. Begin now to make demands upon your muscles by doing both aerobic and weight bearing exercise (see Get Strong). Nice and easy especially if you are not used to it. Not only will your muscles grow stronger and smoother, your bone tissue will become denser.

WHAT'S YOUR BIOAGE?

Researchers investigating the causes of premature ageing and degeneration have come up with objective, easily measurable *biomarkers* of ageing and health. These are scientific measures of how old you are *biologically* not *chronologically*. Forget the birthdays. This is the only age that matters. Making lifestyle changes – Radiance Eating coupled with strength training – can reverse not only how old you look and feel but how your body functions in *medically measurable ways*. Here are the top ten biomarkers. What surprises most people is that lean body mass leads the list. It is the single most important thing in determining how old you are biologically.

TOP TEN BIOMARKERS
Radiance Eating Plus Strength Training Rejuvenates All

- Lean Body Mass
- Muscle Strength
- Basal Metabolic Rate (BMR)
- Body Fat Percentage
- Aerobic Capacity
- Insulin Sensitivity/Blood Sugar Tolerance
- Cholesterol HDL/LDL Ratios
- Blood Pressure
- Bone Density
- Body Heat

POWERFUL DUO

Radiance Eating coupled with strength training transforms your body and your life thanks to two essential actions: One, it re-establishes good insulin/glucose balance so that your body creates energy for itself instead of storing it as fat; two, it builds lean body mass thanks to both its demand for adequate levels of the best protein foods available and because simple strength training exercise improves your lean-to-fat ratio. This significantly reverses your biological age in medically measurable ways.

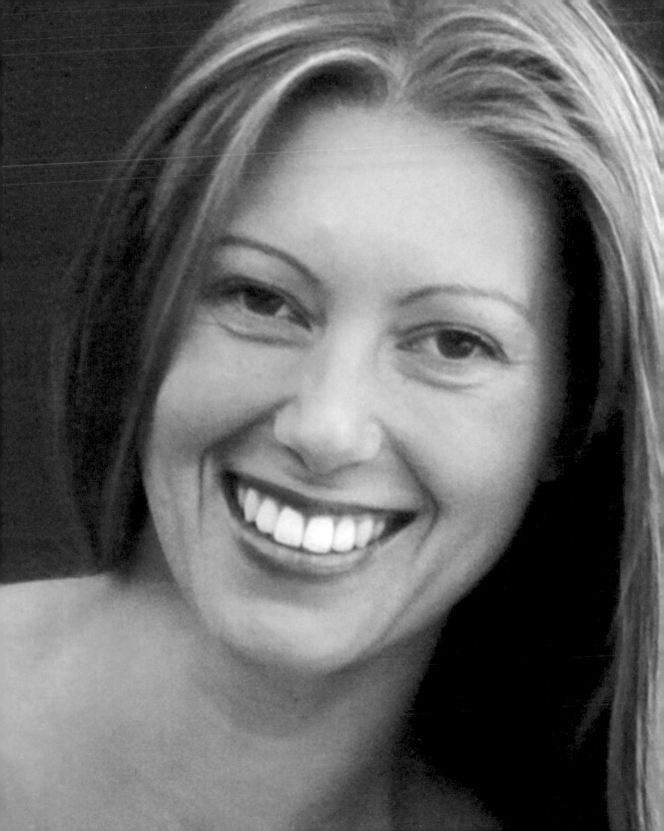

CALL TO ACTION

Cut Cravings: Try the 'glass of water when you feel hungry' approach. For even more support, invest in some L-glutamine to curb appetite.

Snack On: Don't be afraid to eat between meals if you are hungry. Check out the snacks on p.108 and make sure you always have one or two to hand.

Flex Your Muscle: Dive into Get Strong and get started on a strength-training program that can help you muscle-up, burn off excess fat and get healthy and lean for life.

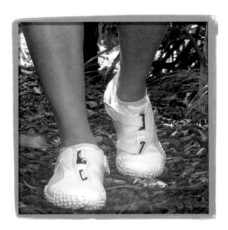

'As you go the way of life, you will
see a great chasm. Jump. It is
not as wide as you think.'
Joseph Campbell

9 GET STRONG
muscle-up and cry

Becoming stronger doesn't mean sacrificing female allure. Nor does it mean developing a tough attitude or a mean karate chop. Real strength is having the courage to live your truth – honouring equally your power and your vulnerability. It brings a priceless confidence that no matter what challenge you may face, you will be more than equal to it.

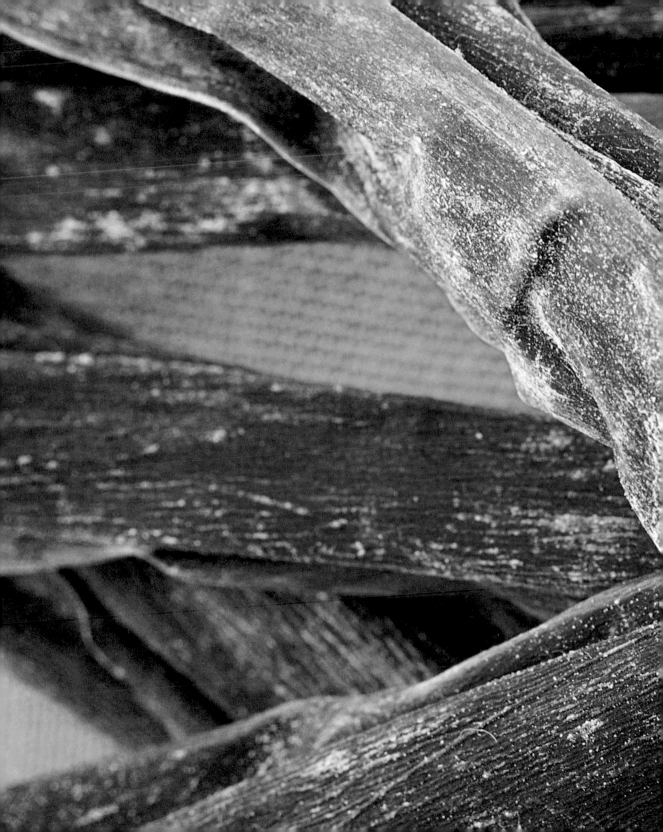

'To me old age is always fifteen years older than I am.'
Bertrand Baruch

We believe there's no better way to develop physical, mental and emotional strength than weight training. Done regularly and *consciously* as an integral practice, resistance training transforms your body on every level. It improves your state of health and creates a solid sense of your own being that makes you glow with self-confidence. It eliminates excess fat and helps to sculpt your body's true form. It also gives you vast reserves of energy and stamina. And you can notice a difference fast – even in a matter of weeks. Instead of struggling helplessly with heavy suitcases or bags of groceries, you find yourself lifting them with ease. Things that once felt like just too much of an effort, like running back upstairs for the second or third time to fetch something you forgot, become as effortless as shrugging your shoulders.

REVERSE AGEING

In 2001, Leslie demonstrated the effect of weight training (combined with a healthy diet and a daily walk) on reversing the signs of age-related degeneration in medically measurable ways. Her documentary *To Age or Not to Age* made television history in the Southern Hemisphere where it aired. Eight men and women between the ages of 30 and 60 were asked to train with weights four times a week. In just four weeks, all eight participants had normalized or dramatically improved their biomarkers – the scientific measurements for age that include parameters like blood pressure, fasting insulin and cholesterol levels.

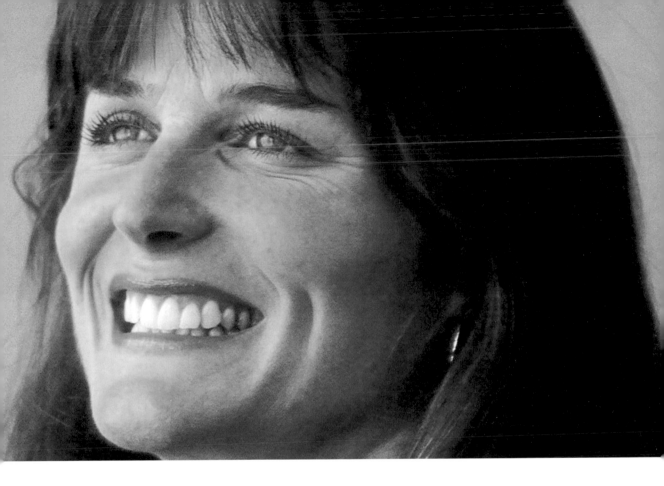

Studies from around the world confirm the impact of weight training on health, strength, rejuvenation and self confidence. Researchers at Tokyo University measured the effects of a 12-week weight-training program on strength. Participants in the study were asked to train three times a week. Their program consisted of just six exercises, each performed for one set of 8-12 repetitions. Even with this relatively light program, by the end of the study, the men taking part had increased their strength by 19 per cent and the women had increased theirs by 23 per cent. Another study, published in the *British Journal of Sports Medicine* put elderly women through a one-year weight-training program. The women showed a 19 to 29 per cent increase in strength, as well as an increase in bone density. Strength training, more than any other form of exercise, does something magical to the muscle in your body.

MITOCHONDRIA BOOST

How much energy you have depends on the numbers of mitochondria (or energy factories) in your cells, which store useable energy as ATP. With age and inactivity, mitochondria function declines by as much as 50 per cent. Strength training boosts mitochondria numbers and activity, helping to restore youthful vitality.

GOOD SEX – FIRM SKIN

Muscle is living, metabolically active tissue. It turns calories and stored fat into useable energy and provides physical and emotional strength. The greater your body's percentage of muscle tissue in relation to fat, the better metabolism functions, the more easily you burn fat and the stronger you feel. Enhancing the quality and mass of your muscle also increases the level of anti-ageing protection you carry, improves your production and balance of sex hormones and firms your skin.

Unlike muscle, fat tissue does not need oxygen, does not create movement and cannot repair itself. Body fat is about as close as you can get to dead flesh within a living system. As resistance training expert Dr Vince Quas says, 'Your lean body mass *is* you, your fat is *on* you.' Reducing excess body fat and increasing lean mass by building muscle increases your body's strength and aliveness.

With age, your proportion of muscle to fat tissue usually declines. Inactive women may lose half a pound of muscle each year, and even more after menopause. The average American woman between the ages of 20 and 40 loses 8 pounds of muscle and gains 23 pounds of fat. The good news is that weight training and consuming adequate quantities of good-quality protein can reverse this decline, helping you achieve quantum health.

Building Strength

The beauty of weight training is how fast your strength can grow. You can invest in several sets of weights or choose adjustable dumbbells to change the weight as needed. What follows is a beginner's routine of standard strength-training exercises, similar to the one Susannah began with. It calls for just dumbbells. It is important to do the exercises with correct form. If you have no experience with weights, we recommend investing in a book and/or DVD/video to help learn the basics (see Resources). You can also hire a good personal trainer to teach you correct form and get you started on a customized weight-training program.

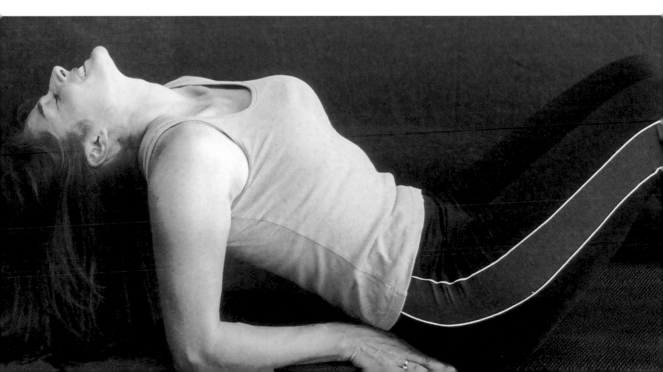

beginner's routine

CHEST/BACK

Dumbbell Flyes (lying on back on the floor, or ideally on a bench.)

Dumbbell Bench Press (lying on back on floor, or ideally on a bench.)

Modified Press-ups (with knees touching floor, ankles crossed. It may take a while to work up to a full set of 12 reps.)

One Arm Row (using a chair to balance opposite knee and hand on. Doing both sides counts as one set.)

Prone Back Extension (lying on stomach, arms by sides. Rotate arms outward, shoulders back, then raise and lower torso.)

Abs Workout (Crunch, Reverse Crunch, Oblique Crunch.)

LEGS

Alternate Lunges (with dumbbells held at sides – each lunge counts as one rep)

Alternate Step-Ups (using a stair or step, with dumbbells held at shoulders – stepping up and back down counts as one rep)

Pliés (feet 2 –3 feet apart, toes comfortably turned out, dumbbells held on upper thighs.)

Leg Abduction (lying on side, raise upper leg 45 degrees and lower – no dumbbells. As you get stronger, add 5lb ankle weights for extra resistance.)

Leg Adduction (lying on side, supporting weight on elbow. Bend upper leg, foot to floor, knee to ceiling. Raise front leg 45 degrees off floor and lower – no dumbbells. As you get stronger, add 5lb ankle weights for extra resistance.)

Abs Workout (Crunch, Reverse Crunch, Oblique Crunch.)

SHOULDERS/ARMS

Standing Lateral Raises

Overhead Press (alternating right and left arm. Each press counts as one rep.)

Standing Upright Row

Biceps Curl (alternating right and left arm. Each curl counts as one rep.)

Triceps Kick Back (doing both arms counts as one set.)

Abs Workout (Crunch, Reverse Crunch, Oblique Crunch.)

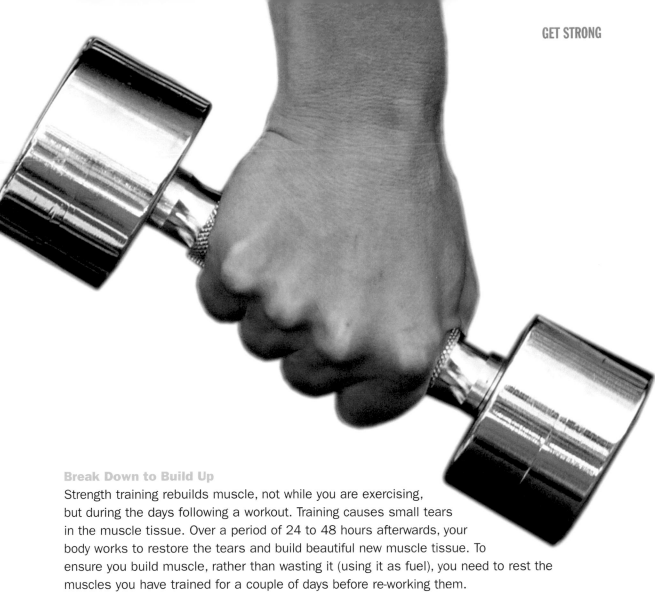

Break Down to Build Up

Strength training rebuilds muscle, not while you are exercising, but during the days following a workout. Training causes small tears in the muscle tissue. Over a period of 24 to 48 hours afterwards, your body works to restore the tears and build beautiful new muscle tissue. To ensure you build muscle, rather than wasting it (using it as fuel), you need to rest the muscles you have trained for a couple of days before re-working them.

The programme opposite is a split routine that focuses on three different groups of muscles. By doing one session every other day, you can complete a full body workout in a week and at the same time give your muscles ample time for recovery.

'Thank you for calling the Weight Loss Hotline. If you'd like to lose a half pound right now, press one 18,000 times.'

Randy Glasbergen

Ease into Power

We have discovered that you don't need a lot of fancy equipment to enjoy the rewards of strength training. A couple of dumbbells will do fine. If necessary, you can even use household objects in place of dumbbells, like a pair of heavy work boots or tins of food. Done correctly, free weight exercises can give you a better workout than many of the expensive machines you find in gyms. That's because free weights (such as dumbbells, barbells and ankle weights) allow full range of motion and call into play stabilizing muscles, which improve balance.

> 'You're a dangerous woman.'
> 'Thanks. You look good to me, too.'
> **Paul Cavanagh and Mae West,** *Goin' to Town*

When choosing dumbbells, do a simple dumbbell curl to find the right weight for you. Hold the weight by your side, palm up, and raise it towards your shoulder, bending your elbow. You should be able to repeat this 12 times, or – in weight-training jargon – complete one set of 12 reps, with the last couple of reps feeling somewhat challenging. If you are struggling at 5 or 6, you need a lighter weight. If doing 12 reps is a breeze, you need to go heavier.

PRIME THOSE MUSCLES

Set aside 20 to 30 minutes for each workout session. Before beginning, we do 5 – 10 minutes of aerobic activity to get the blood circulating and warm up our muscles. We then walk, jog in place, jump rope, row on a machine or rebound. We follow this with a few minutes of gentle stretching to prepare the muscles for exertion and help prevent injury, paying particular attention to the muscle groups we will be working out. If you find some muscles are especially tight, try this trick: inhale, contracting the tight muscle, then exhale as you relax and stretch it. Repeat this sequence several times, working each stretch for about a minute. (While resting between reps we have also learnt that it's also a good idea to stretch the specific muscles being trained.)

Remember to breathe out when you are lifting the weight (or exerting effort) and breathe in as you return to the starting position. You'll get the most benefit from your workout if you raise and lower your weights slowly, taking 3 – 5 seconds to complete each rep. Working with weights is like meditation. Only the muscle group you are working in a particular set is moving. The rest of your body (and mind) is centred, quiet and still. Take about a minute between sets to stretch and recuperate.

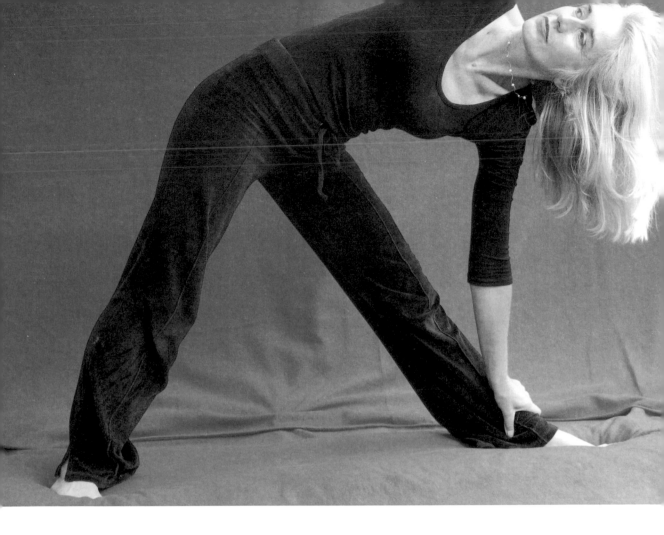

Once our workout is complete, we do a more thorough stretch. The body is warm and muscles are full of blood. Stretching at this point can help flush toxins, lengthen muscles and reduce post-workout soreness.

SOOTHE THE ACHES

Your muscles are likely to ache a little following a weights workout – especially the second day. It is a natural response to the microscopic tears that take place in the muscle tissue and the swelling that accompanies them. If necessary, take a warm Epsom salts bath or sauna/steam bath to ease the discomfort.

INTEGRAL TRANSFORMATIVE POWER

We don't think we have ever come across a more innovative and exciting tool in the realm of health, fitness and strength than the new Power Plate. It is the first truly integral device ever invented for total body treatment. At the cutting-edge of vibrational technology, this space-age instrument helps people reach high levels of fitness in the minimum time. The Power Plate consists of a body positioning plate on which you work out, or simply sit. The plate produces a vibration that is transferred to the body. The vibration magnifies reflexive muscle contraction and in the process improves everything from circulation and lymphatic drainage to your hormone balance. Adjustable in terms of both frequency and amplitude, the Power Plate – which was until recently only used by top athletes to enhance performance – is rightly being hailed as a powerful tool for rehabilitation and as a medical treatment for injury and chronic conditions. Its applications by no means end there. At some frequencies and amplitudes the machine is used for deep relaxation since it can lower cortisol levels and improve your body's ability to handle stress. Used together with the Radiance Diet it helps clear cellulite and brings about significant and *healthy* weight loss. It enhances sports training and performance. It improves the production of Human Growth Hormone and overall hormone balance which makes it an anti-ageing tool. It helps reverse osteoporosis, it even improves brain functions. And you only need use it for 10 – 15 minutes at a time to benefit from its use. The Power Plate is beginning to appear in top gyms and salons. If you haven't tried it, give it a go.

CONSCIOUS MUSCLES

Since we became weight-training enthusiasts nearly two decades ago, we have come to believe that when you work out with awareness and intent you build consciousness into your tissues. Your intention could be as simple as to sculpt your true form. Or it might be to harness your personal power. This is another way in which the diverse practices in this book are integral to your journey towards becoming more authentic.

By focusing your mind as you work your muscles, you build the vibration of who you are and what you believe into your body. You then carry that with you wherever your authentic path may lead.

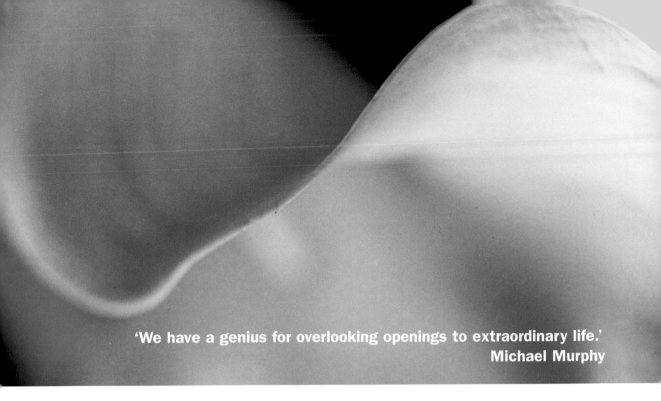

'We have a genius for overlooking openings to extraordinary life.'
Michael Murphy

Try dedicating a weight-training session to something you'd like to create – a lean, beautiful body, a new relationship, a business venture. Focus on your intention and use it to drive your muscular exertion. Whatever feelings come up in relation to your goal – anger, fear, excitement – use them as fuel. Combining the power of your mind and muscle will help ground your vision in your body.

TRANSCENDENTAL TRAINING

Karen Andes, American expert in weight training for women, describes the experience of reaching muscle failure. (This is where muscles feel so tired you cannot do another rep.)

'You can no longer continue without cheating, so you just hold the weight, hanging out here on the edge, biting down in the jaw, coaxing one more fibre and the moment stretches out like a desert. You want to drop the weight and scream but instead, lower it with the exquisite sensitivity of a mother laying down the head of her newborn...'

Protein Strengthens All Round

To build strong, beautiful muscles, you need to make sure you replenish your body's protein supply daily. Every molecule of muscle in your body is made from the protein-containing foods you eat. One half of the dry weight of your body – that is when water is removed – is protein. If you improve the quality, that is the biological value, of your proteins and get enough in your diet, you can completely transform, regenerate and rejuvenate how your body functions as well as how you look.

SUNSHINE MAKES YOU STRONGER

Adequate sun exposure is important – at every age. Exposing skin to sunshine increases the amount of vitamin D your body produces. Higher concentrations of vitamin D can bolster muscle strength and function. Roman gladiators knew this well. They trained naked in the sun to build strength. You can boost your own vitamin D levels and muscle strength by stripping down and weight training in the sun.

Meat and fish, which we've always been told are the top-quality proteins, are actually lower in biological value than the best protein sources. One form of protein, still known only to an élite group of athletes and health seekers, is heads above the rest. It's called micro-filtered whey or ion-exchange whey. There's nothing like micro-filtered or ion-exchange whey to build muscle fast and bring about cell renewal. It improves skin, strengthens arteries and helps reshape your whole body. MFW does wonderful things for your immune system, too, thanks to its active ingredients called subfractions. It is one of the few processed foods where technology has been used to enhance the health-creating powers of nature. We use it all the time, blended with pure water or soy milk and a handful of berries, for a quick breakfast, lunch on-the-go, or as a post-workout snack. We love the strength it brings on every level.

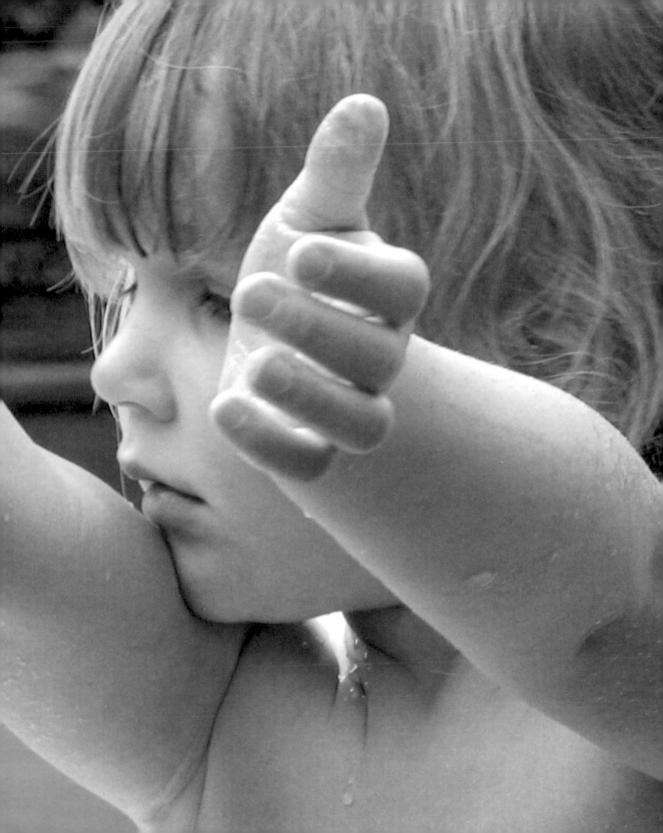

Freedom To Be

As women we are often urged to 'be strong'. You know the rhetoric. 'Pull yourself together.' 'Dry your tears.' 'Don't let your feelings show.' Whether struggling for equality in the workplace or maintaining our integrity in relationships, the implication is that feelings and tears are signs of weakness.

We disagree. A woman's true strength doesn't come from steeling herself against adversity or putting on a brave face. Real strength is the ability to show up *as you are* – even when that's tearful, angry or messy. Only when we allow ourselves the freedom to be completely who we are do we move fully into strength and power at every level of our being. And that's not power *over* anyone, but the power to effect positive change in our lives and the lives of others – the power to envision what we want to create and make it happen. Pretending to be strong never brings this. Being real, and consciously choosing to develop strength can.

TEARS OF GRACE

Scientists have identified three kinds of tears: basal, which provide lubrication, reflex, which are produced in response to irritation, and emotional. Tears cried for emotional reasons differ from the others in that they have a higher composition of chemicals, including ACTH – an adrenal stress hormone. Researchers, including Dr. William Frey at the Ramsay Medical Center, Minnesota, believe that chemicals excreted in emotional tears soothe us by helping the body release stress hormones. You know from experience how much better you can feel after a good cry. So let your tears flow when they need to and trust them.

'...living in strength gives us no need to wear armour, but the courage to reveal ourselves as we are.'

Karen Andes

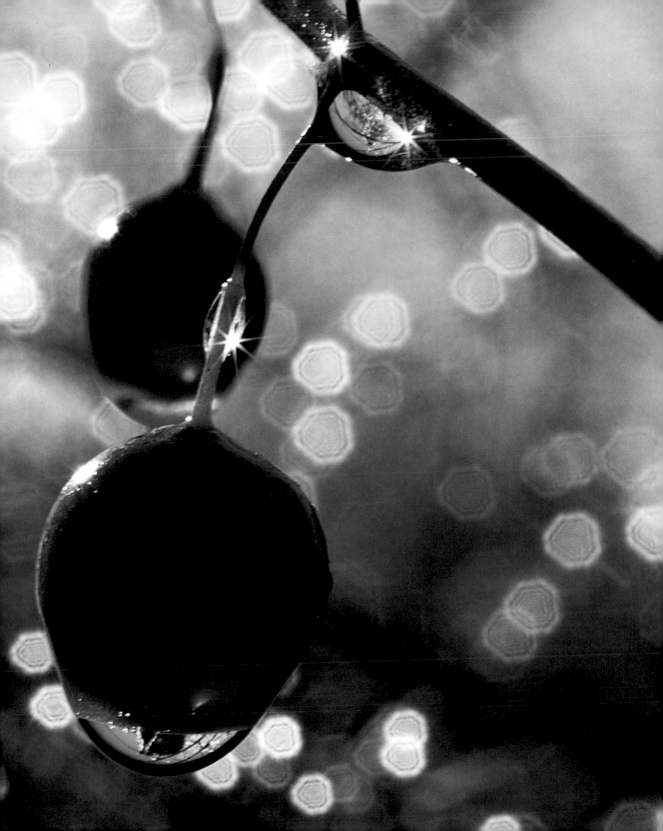

CALL TO ACTION

Pump Some Iron: Get yourself a set of dumbbells and begin to discover for yourself the strength and renewal that come from weight training. Offer yourself a handful of sessions with a personal trainer to get you started, or find a friend who is savvy with weights and get them to coach you through the exercises in the beginner's program.

Power Shake: Create your own delicious smoothie recipes using micro-filtered whey. Try rice or soy milk blended with chocolate or vanilla protein powder and fresh or frozen raspberries, blueberries, banana or mango.

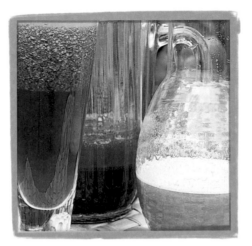

'To know consists in opening out a way
Whence the imprisoned splendour may escape.'
Robert Browning

10 NO COMPROMISE
create win-win relationships

We long for relationships because we long for union. We want connection and nourishment. We want to share our strength, our aliveness with others – to inspire and to be inspired. To experience the heights and depths of feeling and bask in the warmth of true friendship. Authentic, alive, satisfying relationships with others are only possible when you relate authentically to yourself first – right from your very soul.

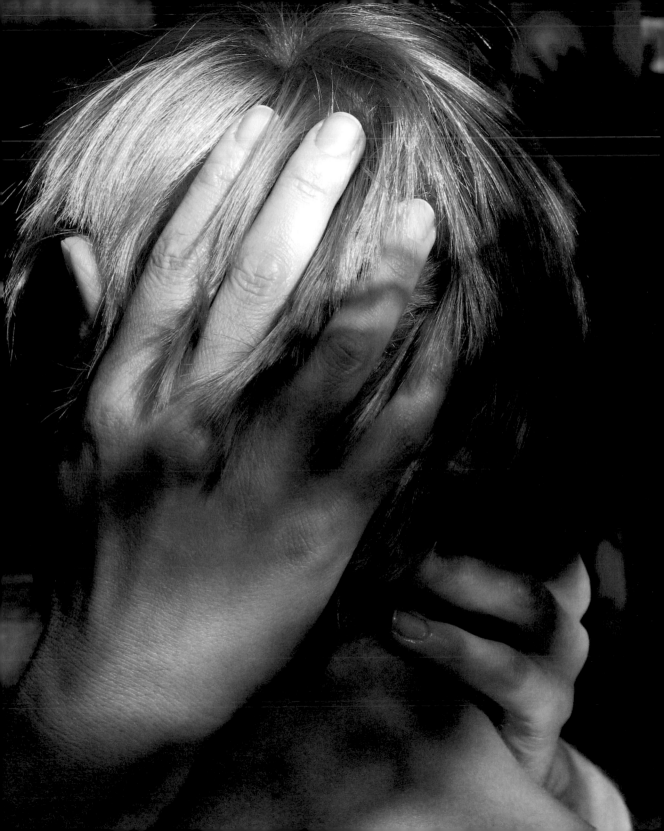

It is the nature of every man, woman and child to expand, to explore, to celebrate life and to express oneself. Too often, however, as our core energy flows forth, it gets blocked. Why? In a small part because we pick up a lot of misguided notions as we grow up. They come from parental training, from religion, from school. Then, unbeknown to us, they become part of our belief system, our worldview, and limit our lives in a thousand ways.

SCRUB THE BRAINWASHING

Without realizing it, we bring these notions to the relationship table. Once there, they interfere with our ability to connect authentically person to person, soul to soul. 'I should always be kind,' 'I mustn't say what I really think' or 'I might hurt her feelings.' 'Men are self-centred.' 'Women have to stand up for themselves.' 'Marriage is forever.' Our distorted views and expectations get foisted onto others, creating all sorts of 'shoulds' and 'shouldn'ts' for us and them. Then, when in relationships our expectations are not met, we can fall into the familiar bitching or whining of which women are so often accused: 'If you really loved me you would…' 'You never listen.' You know the drill. Under such pressure even the best relationship can turn sour and become frustrating, deadening, or full of grief. This doesn't have to happen so long as you get the most important relationship in your life right: the relationship with *yourself*.

The only way to relate honestly to friends, children, lovers, workmates, even pets, is to honour yourself at the deepest possible level first. When you do – and it's got to be *real*, you can't fake this – you open yourself to a universe of unprecedented vitality, satisfaction, excitement and connections with other people that really work.

You begin to experience the kind of connections with others that *do not* bind. Instead, they free the spirits of all involved. Rules and regulations dissolve to be replaced by a directness, honesty and vitality so satisfying that you wonder why you ever chose roles, rules and obligations in the first place.

> 'To love oneself is the beginning of a life-long romance.'
> Oscar Wilde

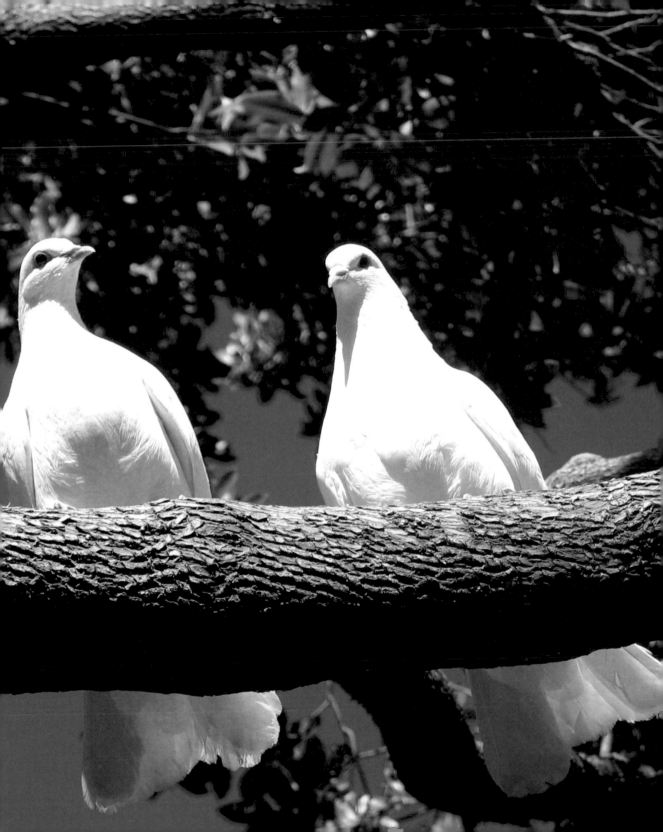

The Art of Self-Nurturing

As women, our genes have been encoded to nurture others. It's a biological inheritance that ensures the survival of the species. Caring for *ourselves* can feel foreign. Self-sacrifice is a familiar path. Yet looking after yourself well is a necessity for your own personal evolution, and also if you are to be able to nurture others properly. It builds a solid foundation for every relationship in life. It allows us to shift out of burn-out mode so that we don't just get through each day, we savour it. Let's play with some integral processes that can help expand relationships, both to self and to others.

How do you express love for a partner? Do you listen and reassure them when times are tough? Massage them? Write encouraging notes? Offer gifts? Prepare delicious food?

Pick up your Journal and make a list of things you frequently do for your partner, children or friends. Then look at how you might start redirecting some of those expressions of love to yourself.

For instance:

- **I take my children to the zoo.** I could take myself to the zoo/a concert/the theatre.
- **I take my mother flowers whenever I visit.** I could give myself a bouquet of flowers.
- **I listen to my partner rant about his work day.** I could tell a friend about my day or listen to myself. Proprioceptive Writing is a good way to do this.

If you could really see who you were, you couldn't help but fall in love with yourself. The soul of each of us is spectacularly beautiful. When you practise acts of self-nurturing, your love for yourself naturally grows. You can accelerate the process by going within and connecting with who you are at the soul level.

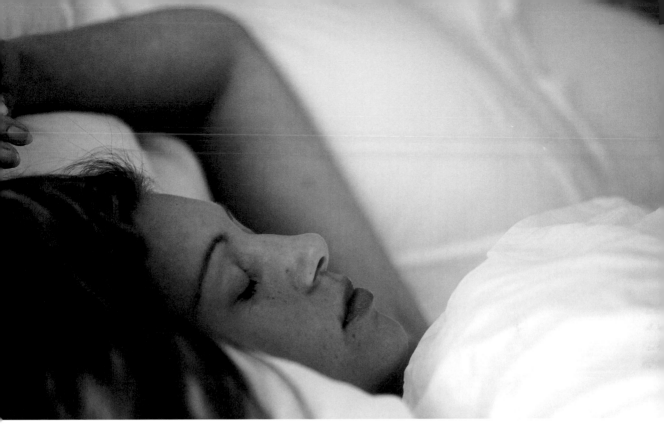

JUST FOR FUN

Many women feel guilty when they take time to care for their needs. If this sounds familiar, make a practice of doing something nurturing for yourself each day, or at least once a week. Take it seriously. Keep a list of activities so you have plenty to choose from. Here are a few of our favourites:

- Get a massage or some form of delicious bodywork.
- Watch a fun movie.
- Spend the morning in bed – or even the whole day.
- Take a bath or a sauna.
- Visit an art exhibition.
- Go water-skiing.
- Listen to an audio book.
- Talk on the phone with an old friend.

date with your soul

Here's an inner journey that helps awaken unconditional love for yourself. You might want to record it or have a friend read it aloud. Be sure to leave plenty of time at the ellipses (30 to 60 seconds or so, go by feel) for the images to develop.

Sit in a chair or lie down. Get comfortable. Close your eyes and relax. Breathe softly. As you exhale, feel yourself releasing any cares or concerns… Let any tension in your body melt away… Now imagine a ball of sunlight in your solar plexus… Sense the warmth and peace it brings… Watch the ball become brighter and gradually expand outwards, until your entire body is filled with light… Feel yourself floating in a sea of light… Now imagine you are gradually being lifted up, higher and higher, beyond space and time… In this special place, call forth your divine blueprint – the energy of your soul… Invite your blueprint to enter through the crown of your head and fill your entire body… Feel its energy flooding each of your cells… Bask in the bliss… Let your body overflow with unconditional love… Savour it… When you are ready, gently bring your awareness back to the contact between your physical body and the surface you are sitting or lying on… In your own time, open your eyes.

EXTENDING LOVE TO OTHERS

When you nurture yourself, it gets easier to love those around you. Even your attitude to people who once irritated you begins to soften. You find yourself naturally spending more time in love than in judgment. That's not to say that every relationship in your life becomes blissful and trouble-free. But the blessings your relationships bring become more apparent and more abundant.

JUST SAY IT

Saying 'yes' to someone when you want to say 'no' cripples authenticity. Learning to say 'no' can set you free. At first it feels scary. You worry about hurting feelings or losing love. Later on you come to realize that saying 'no' to another is usually saying 'yes' to yourself. Practise using the 'N' word, without needing to apologize or make excuses. Begin where the stakes are small, then graduate to more significant situations.

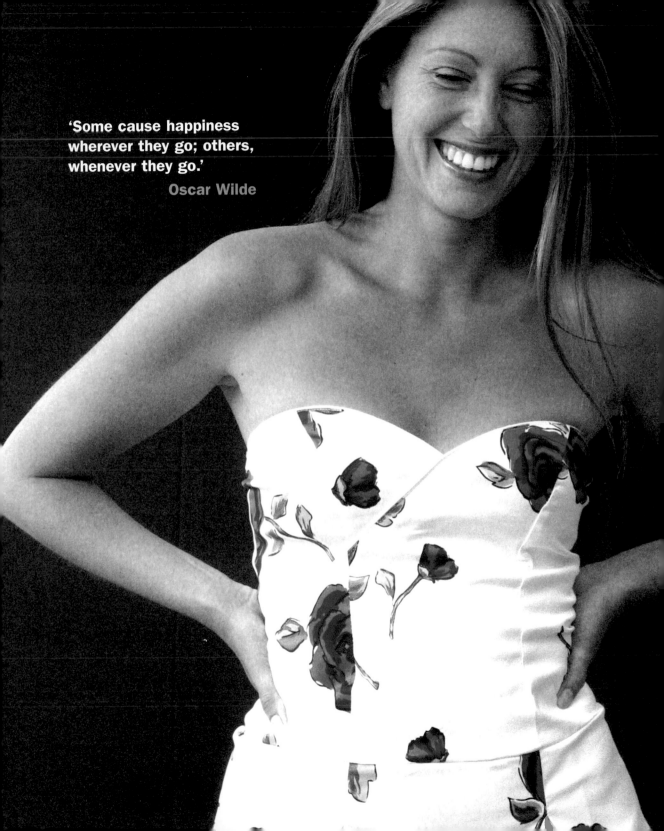

'Some cause happiness
wherever they go; others,
whenever they go.'
Oscar Wilde

A Fine Romance

Disappointment, betrayal, heartbreak. For women they are all-too-common outcomes of romantic relationships. The assumption is 'a good man is hard to find' (let alone the prodigious 'handsome prince' of girlhood programming). We can spend decades in the quest for 'the one' only to discover, when he arrives then lets us down, that he wasn't the one after all. As women we have choice. We can go on blaming men and feeling like victims, or we can create a new framework for intimate relationships.

In the old model for romantic relationships and marriage, you commit yourself to one person, no matter what, for life. For a few, it seems to work. Divorce statistics suggest, however, that it may not be the ultimate pathway for many to find happiness and fulfilment.

The new model for love invites you to commit to the process of deepening your intimacy *with yourself* through your relationship. You see your relationship with a significant other not as an end in itself but as something in the service of your unfolding – and theirs.

The new model for love means that, whether you stay together for life – you well may – or discover after a few years that your relationship has run its course and you decide to separate, the experience is still 'a success'. The process of separation can be as enriching as coming together.

HOW CAN YOU TELL IF IT'S LOVE?

'If in your relationships you experience both "love" and the opposite of love – attack, emotional violence, and so on – then it is likely that you are confusing ego attachment and addictive clinging with love.'

Eckhart Tolle

'Every important relationship I have ever had has awakened me to a new way of looking at life and brought me in touch with parts of myself I did not know existed. Exciting, challenging, sometimes painful, always different, the process of intimacy has been one of the most transformative in my life. Most often that process in relation to a particular man has completed itself, bringing the relationship to a close in its own time and its own way. Then either the man who was once my lover becomes a life-long friend or like as not I never see him again.'

Leslie

The new model for love also calls for autonomy. Instead of surrendering self-responsibility and setting up expectations of what your partner should do to support you, it invites you to be self-sustaining – to find ways to support yourself. This frees both partners from games of control and manipulation that cloud the simple pleasure of loving and being loved. It allows for a more genuine connection where couples love and support one another not out of obligation but for the joy of it.

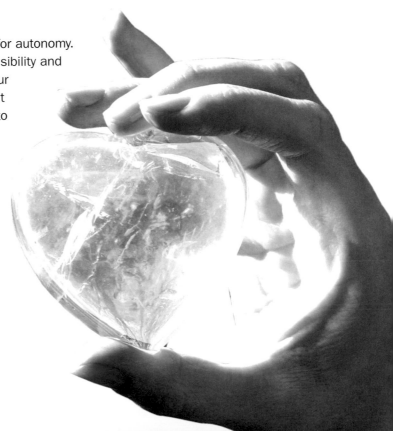

ON THE SAME SEXUAL WAVELENGTH

The battle of the sexes is often fought and lost by both sides in the bedroom. Making love is an unequalled way of touching the depths of your soul, merging with the oneness of the divine and experiencing the bliss that is your birthright. Couples can miss out on the wonder and possibilities of sexual union when hidden agendas prevent them from connecting fully. Sexual energy is powerful. Like a full moon, it magnifies whatever is in your consciousness. If you begin to make love with underlying anger or resentment then that, rather than feelings of love, will be amplified.

The following exercise, taken from the Tantric tradition, is deceptively simple and yet highly effective. It helps clear the obstacles to intimacy, creating a space for bliss to enter. Use it when you need to clear the air. It can be especially rewarding if lovemaking has become routine and predictable. It helps you and your partner to rediscover the excitement of getting to know one another again, as if for the first time.

'When the authorities warn you of the dangers of having sex, there is an important lesson to be learned. Do not have sex with the authorities.'

Matt Groening

MAKE YOUR BED BEFORE YOU LIE IN IT

Set aside time when you won't be disturbed. Prepare a 'sanctuary' in which to make love. Make sure you are comfortable and have whatever you need – cushions, something to drink, towels, massage oil, whatever. Light a candle. Sit comfortably facing your partner. Take a few moments to become still and focused.

Now take turns to express how you are feeling. One person speaks while the other listens with an open heart. It's important for the person listening to be just still and witness what is said without judging or taking anything personally.

The person who is speaking expresses:

● How they are feeling – especially any feelings/fears/desires about making love.

● Anything they feel might be standing in the way of connecting intimately.

● What they love about their partner.

The first person speaks for as long as necessary until they feel clear. For example, he or she might begin:

OK, let's see… I'm feeling a bit awkward about this process, but I really want to deepen our connection. I feel so much love and desire for you that sometimes I don't know how to express it. The last time we made love I felt a bit rushed. I also had the sense that you were trying hard to please me and I felt like I needed to show you that you were pleasing me, but in doing so I somehow lost the sense of who I was. I'd like to throw away the rules – expectations about orgasm – and just explore each other's body in a new way…

Then reverse the roles. The second person speaks while the first listens. The process can continue back and forth until all agendas have been cleared. At this point, according to the Tantric tradition, each partner bows to the god/goddess in the other and lovemaking begins. The scene has been set for heightened intimacy, spontaneity and pleasure. Let it take you where it may.

TROUBLESHOOT RELATIONSHIPS

While relationships can be the source of our greatest joy, they can also trigger our most intense heartache. An unresolved, angst-ridden relationship, such as to a parent or an ex-lover you feel wronged by, can cloud your ability to experience love and joy for years.

Fortunately there are tools you can use to dissolve the shackles of resentment, pain, injustice or disillusion you feel in relation to another and to set yourself free. One very good one is Byron Katie's *The Work*. A process of self-inquiry, The Work involves four questions and a 'turn-around'. It is a useful way to unravel the pain and stress we experience in relation to anyone or anything by questioning our thoughts and discovering the deeper truth. Susannah once watched Katie, the creator of the process, do The Work with a gay man whose lover had hanged himself a year earlier. The man was filled with despair and anger that his lover had chosen to take his life. He continued to be haunted by the image of discovering the hanged body. Katie took him through the inquiry process and then invited him, in his imagination, to go back to the scene when he had found his dead lover. As he did, the man began to laugh. For the first time he saw the event without his 'story' attached to it. In that moment he became free from the heartbreak he had carried for a year. To learn how to use The Work for yourself, read *Loving What Is – Four Questions That Can Change Your Life* by Byron Katie and Stephen Mitchell, published by Harmony Books. Or you can go online to www.thework.org to find out about it.

BEAR WITNESS

When relationships get tough, we may have a tendency to shut down and avoid contact. We fear that our state of anger, grief or depression will drag someone else down and we don't want to be a burden. But although solitude can help us find our way, too much isolation can leave us feeling cut off from everyone and everything. When you are going through difficulties, call on the power of deep listening. Ask a friend to sit with you and do nothing but bear witness to what you are feeling. Relieve them of the burden to advise or try to make you feel better. Ask them simply to listen and be with you, right where you are. We have learned in our own mother-daughter relationship that this witnessing is often a far greater gift than all the positive suggestions in the world.

DARE TO GET REAL

An authentic path invites you to become more and more truthful in the way you relate to everybody in your life – from your lover, to your child, to your bank manager. The more you do, the more you find that each encounter further supports the unfolding of your authenticity. Instead of having to 'put on a brave face' when you feel down, or adjust your behaviour to fit with how you think someone wants you to be, you give yourself permission to show up just as you are. Self-acceptance breeds appreciation. Life expands. In time, the possibilities for enjoying relationships with people, animals, trees and all of creation becomes boundless.

'Everyone is a mirror image of yourself –
your own thinking coming back at you.'

Byron Katie

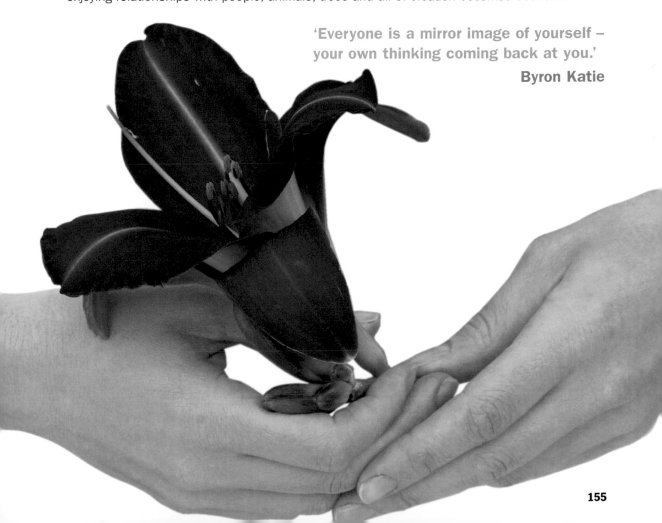

CALL TO ACTION

Art of Self-Nurturing: After making a list of activities you would enjoy that are *all about you*, pick one and make a promise to do it within the next week. No excuses.

A Date With Your Soul: Find a time when you can take the guided inner journey on p.148. If you don't have someone to read it out loud for you, look through the journey a couple of times to familiarize yourself. Once you complete the journey, record your experience in your Journal. Use this journey often to recharge yourself with unconditional love.

Do The Work: If there is a relationship in your life that is upsetting you, try The Work of Byron Katie. You can go online and print out a copy of the worksheet and instructions to get started right away.

Make Your Bed: If you are in a relationship, see whether your partner is willing to explore the Tantric exercise on p.152. Make a date when the night is young or the day is long and *enjoy*.

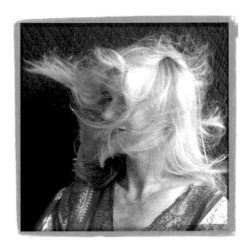

'Only through being yourself can you give to the others in your world your greatest gifts. To do any less betrays both them and yourself.'
Ken Carey

11 SPACEFIX
focus and watch it happen

Like the body itself, the environment in which you live and work carries palpable energy. The energy of a particular space can be conditioned to support health and vitality, to relax you, to energize you, to enhance your ability to create the life you want. Learn to do this through conscious intentions and you can create ideal surroundings for every aspect of your life. Did you ever walk into an office after someone has been fired? Or enter a room in which an argument has just taken place? If so, you'll know first-hand that disruptive energy can linger. On the positive side, you can find yourself in a house, a museum, a cathedral, where the atmosphere is so inviting you just don't want to leave.

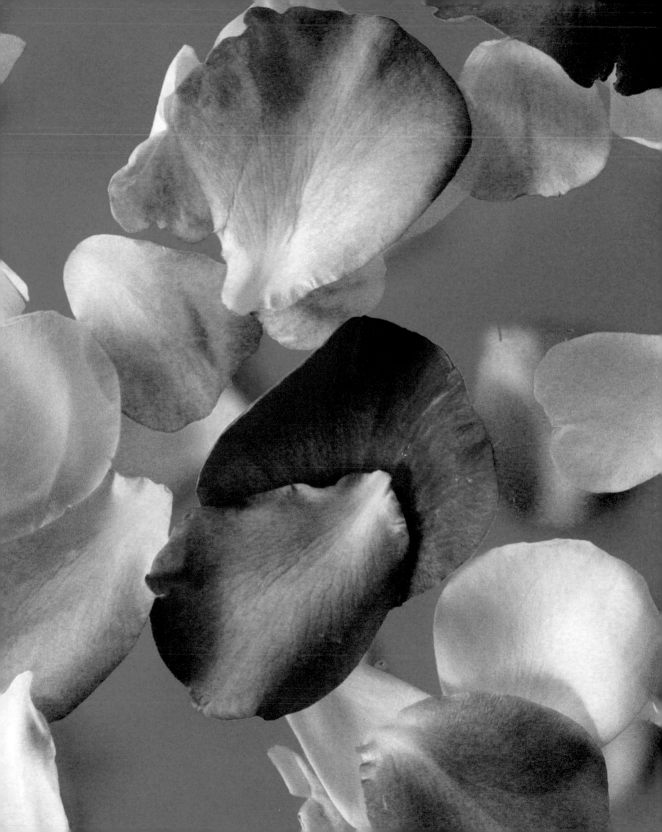

From Magic to Science

The idea that focused human intention – both conscious and unconscious – changes reality once belonged to the realm of the supernatural. No longer. Science cannot yet fully explain how it occurs, but there is plenty of proof that it does. In the past 25 years, well-controlled, university-based studies show clearly that human consciousness significantly alters material reality. We do not just 'stop' at our skin. Our influence extends well beyond that. Studies show that every one of us continually influences the energy of the space in which we live and work, whether we are aware of it or not. We can't help it because of the holographic nature of the universe. The trick is to learn to do it consciously.

'Because of the interconnectedness of all minds, affirming a positive vision may be about the most sophisticated action any one of us can take'.

Willis Harman

PSYCHOENERGETIC POWER

William A. Tiller's work stands out amongst a growing number of paradigm-breaking scientists who map the way human intention alters physical reality. Fellow to the American Academy for the Advancement of Science, and Professor Emeritus of Stanford University's Department of Materials Science, Tiller has a background in semiconductor processing and psychoenergetics (the direct focus of human intentions). He and his team have demonstrated beyond all doubt the power of intention to alter reality.

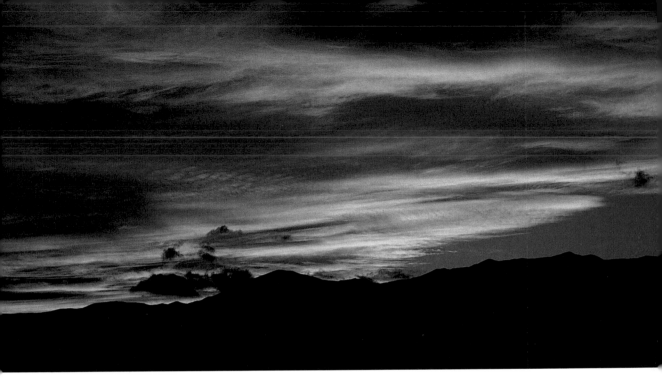

INTEND AND WATCH IT HAPPEN

Tiller conducted research with what he calls 'highly-inner-self-managed' people – people who have trained themselves to expand consciousness and quiet their minds, often through regular meditation. He discovered that when even a handful of such people focus on a specific intention, they are able to shift reality in all sorts of fascinating ways. In one experiment, four people 'imprinted' an electrical device with an intention to alter the pH of water – something previously considered impossible to do. It worked. But Tiller's team then took their experiment further. Researchers wrapped the intention-imprinted electrical device in aluminium foil and shipped it 2,000 miles to another laboratory. In the second lab, researchers reported that when they placed water in the vicinity of the impregnated electrical device the pH was also altered in exactly the same way.

Tiller's real *pièce de résistance* came later. After having repeated these experiments a number of times in the same location, he and his team realised that even the laboratory in which the four 'intentioners' had been focusing had become positively 'conditioned' to alter pH. This meant that the same results would occur more strongly and more rapidly than ever. 'In one of the spaces that we have used,' says Tiller, 'the alteration in the space of the room has remained stable for well over a year and is still going strong.'

SANCTIFYING SPACE

The phenomenon Tiller and his colleagues were studying has been used for centuries by spiritual teachers and meditators to create 'sacred space' – environments that enhance meditation, healing and prayer. What is new and exciting is that experiments by Tiller, as well as many other pioneering researchers, now scientifically validate the way intention can be used to sanctify space.

Energy is everything. Even material forms – dogs, kayaks, grapevines – are nothing but crystallized energy. A physicist would describe the phenomenon by saying that focused consciousness can raise a room's 'physics gauge symmetry'. You don't have to understand physics to put these techniques to work to improve your own life. You can start right now to enhance your health, increase serenity and vitality and create the perfect energetic space in which to do exercise, prepare food, make love, whatever your heart desires.

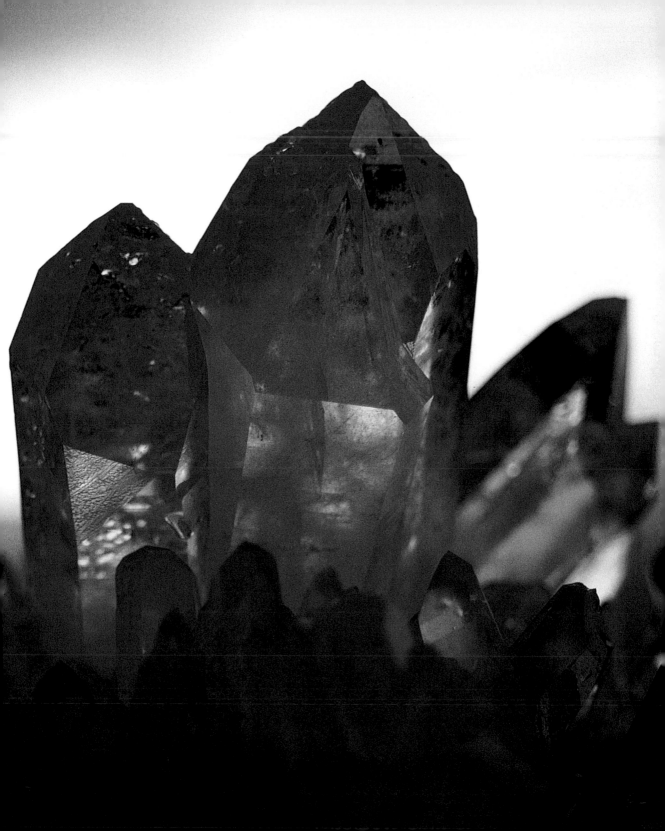

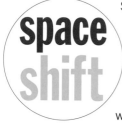

space shift

Space clearing and dedication is designed to remove stagnant or 'negative' energy from a place where you live or work and replace it with positive vibes and conscious intentions to support you on your authentic path. In truth there is no such thing as 'negative energy'. Energy is energy. It only becomes 'negative' when it is in the wrong place. Soil in your garden is a positive thing, for instance, but you don't want it in your bed.

Space clearing is terrific fun. By all means do it on your own, but it makes a great party. Invite friends along, children too – they make excellent drummers – and why not drag the pets along? Make yourselves into a noisy, laughter-filled parade and claim your space with glee.

To transform a living/working space you need to do two things:

● **Open Your Awareness:** You can create this by simply listening to uplifting music, meditating for five minutes, or making a noise yourself – drumming for instance – to let go of day-to-day worries.

● **Create a Simple Intention:** Such as, to clear unhelpful energy and refresh the space.

USE SPACE CLEARING...

● When you move into a new home, apartment or office to get rid of the energy of previous inhabitants.

● After any difficult life change, such as being laid off work, the break-up of a relationship or the death of a loved one.

● After any accident, illness or robbery to clear out unhelpful energies and restore order.

● Whenever you feel stuck in your life and want to make a fresh start.

● At the New Year or as a 'spring cleaning' ritual.

● Whenever there has been unhappiness or conflict in your space.

● When you want to change the purpose for which a particular room is used.

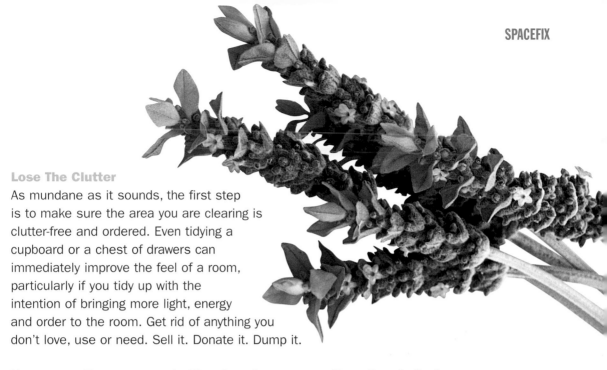

Lose The Clutter

As mundane as it sounds, the first step is to make sure the area you are clearing is clutter-free and ordered. Even tidying a cupboard or a chest of drawers can immediately improve the feel of a room, particularly if you tidy up with the intention of bringing more light, energy and order to the room. Get rid of anything you don't love, use or need. Sell it. Donate it. Dump it.

Now comes the energy work. It's a two-step process. Clear, then dedicate.

Your Tool Kit:

Gather the following space-clearing/dedicating equipment:

- **A Candle (or several)**
- **Matches/A Lighter**
- **A Fireproof Dish**
- **A Ceremonial Cloth (optional)**
- **A Drum or Rattle:** We like Remo shamanic drums, which you can hold in one hand and beat with the other. If you don't have a drum, you can use a rattle. Buy one from a music shop or toyshop, or make your own by filling an empty jar/yoghurt carton with dried beans, peas or seeds.
- **Herbs and Resins:** Native Americans use smudge sticks made from sage, sweetgrass and other herbs for cleansing and ceremony. You can buy smudge sticks ready-made or make your own (see overleaf). You can also use resin incense, or a combination of resin and herbs. We favour copal gold, a resin extracted from the copal tree. The Mayans used copal on altars in sacred ceremonies and considered it so holy they would not touch it with bare hands. You burn copal and other resins on small charcoal briquettes in a fireproof dish. You can add other herbs and resins to it – such as frankincense, sandalwood or lavender. For two millennia, the Catholic Church has used combinations of herbs and resins to sanctify their cathedrals. Church suppliers sell the charcoal you need for burning resin and loose herbs. (They also sell top-quality inexpensive candles.)

MAKE YOUR OWN SMUDGE STICKS

Collect handfuls of herbs. Always harvest growing herbs with respect and gratitude. Good herbs for smudge sticks and incense include: sagebrush, sage, sweetgrass, juniper, eucalyptus, cedar, lavender, mint and rosemary. Arrange the herbs around a central twig or branch. Tie them in a torpedo shape with cotton or embroidery thread. Hang the smudge sticks up for several days until they are dry enough to burn.

● **A Chime** The sound of a Tibetan or Japanese singing bowl, a crystal singing bowl or a beautiful bell, chime or harmony ball, sets a new vibration after you have cleansed a space. (Harmony balls are small metal spheres that make a magical bell-like sound.) If you don't have any of these, you can improvise a chime by tapping lightly on a good-quality glass with a wooden chopstick.

● **Space-Blessing Water:** Make your own 'holy water' using a plant spritzer filled with pure water and fragranced with the essential oils of your choice (see p.171). Holy water, by the way, is just water that has been blessed with an intention.

GORGEOUS AND FUN

It's easy to make your own blessing water. Fill a clean, pint-sized, plant spray bottle with pure water. Add your essential oils. About 12 – 18 drops combined gives you a potent room spray. Then put in 1 drop of washing-up liquid as an emulsifier and give it a good shake. Be sure to use only the best-quality oils, never synthetics (see Resources).

● **Salt:** Useful for ridding a space of stubborn energies, rock salt or sea crystals work best. (You'll also need a number of little dishes to contain it.)

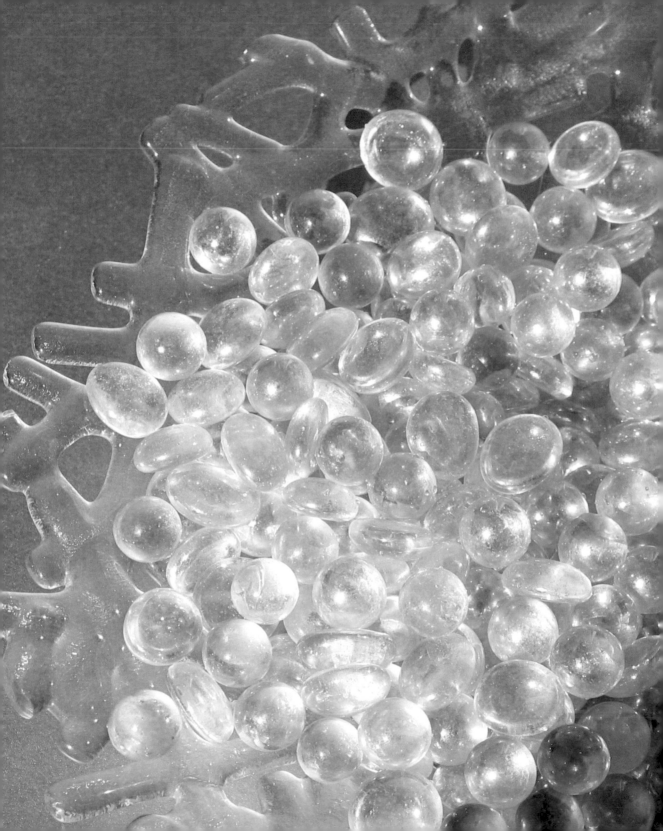

STEP ONE: CLEARING

Light a candle. Focus your intention to clear the space. You can call in the support of spirit helpers if you wish. These may be the people you meet in the Inner Reaches of Sacred Space – guardian angels, power animals, nature divas, spiritual teachers or guides. You can also call in the powers of the six directions – East, South, West, North, Above and Below.

'Honour all with whom we share the Earth: four-leggeds, two-leggeds, winged ones, swimmers, crawlers, plant and rock people. Walk in balance and beauty.'

Native American Elder

Drum Up a Storm

Start with the first room you want to clear. Drum, rattle or clap your hands loudly while holding the intention firmly in your mind to clear out all stagnant energy. Move around the room, paying special attention to the corners where old energy accumulates like cobwebs. Your drum, rattle or clapping may have a slightly muffled sound when you begin. The sound becomes more resonant as the space clears. Children get especially enthusiastic about this part of the ritual if you let them join in.

Once the energy in one room is cleared, go on to the next until all are done. It doesn't matter whether you 'sense' energy easily or not. Keep your intention clear and trust your intuition. You'll know when a room is complete and it is time to move on.

'I think a good way to conceive of sacred space is as a playground. If what you're doing seems like play, you are in it.'

Joseph Campbell

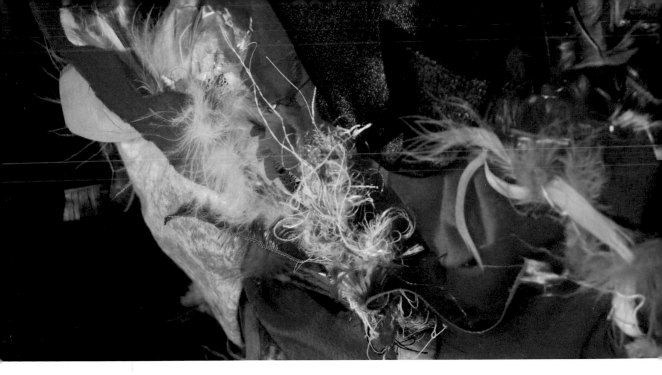

Smoke It Out

Now light your smudge stick or charcoal in a fireproof dish. You may need to carry the dish with an oven glove as it can get very warm. If you use a smudge stick, make sure it is burning well and then blow out the flames so that it smoulders and smokes. (It may need to be relit as you go through the room or rooms.) If you are using charcoal and resin or incense, light the charcoal, and let it burn until it begins to turn grey. Then add your resin and herbs. Walk around your home allowing the smoke to reach into every corner, wafting it with your hand. Be sure to smudge the inside of cupboards and closets too.

PURIFICATION BY SALT

In addition to drumming and smudging, you can also use salt to purify a space, especially if energy in a room feels particularly 'heavy'.

Place a small dish with a handful of sea salt or rock salt in each corner of the room. Set the intention that the salt clear the space. Leave the salt in place for 24 hours, then take it out and bury it in the ground, asking the Earth to transmute and recycle the energy it carries.

STEP TWO: DEDICATION

When you've drummed and smudged each room, you're ready to dedicate. With a singing bowl, bell, harmony balls or glass, stand in the centre of each room and speak a dedication (see suggestions below).

Chime the bowl, bell or glass and allow the sound vibration to carry into every corner. Chiming for about a minute is usually enough.

What's Your Intention?

Here are a few suggestions for different rooms. Use them as inspiration to make up your own.

- **Study:** I intend that my workroom become a place of creativity where I feel clear, focused and connected as I work. I bless this space.
- **Bedroom:** I intend for my bedroom to be a place of relaxation and renewal where I enjoy blissful sleep each night.
- **Living Room:** I bless my living room as a place where all who enter feel welcome. I call in the energies of fun, relaxation, heart-warming community and love to uplift this space.
- **Kitchen:** I bless my kitchen and intend it to become a place where I delight to prepare delicious and healthy meals to nourish myself and others physically, mentally and spiritually.

Finish off the ceremony by spritzing each room with the blessing water you have made. You can use the same fragrance throughout the house or make up a different one for each room. Opposite are some essential oil combinations you can use to support your intentions for different rooms:

ESSENTIAL OILS FOR BLESSING WATER

For concentration	Basil, Rosemary, Lemon Verbena, Hyssop, Neroli
For creativity & vision	Narcissus, Yarrow
For confidence	Melissa, Hyacinth, Rosemary, Rose Otto, Carnation
For relaxation & mental calm	Chamomile, Jasmine, Lavender, Linden Blossom, Clary Sage, Geranium
For mental alertness	Thyme, Rosemary, Jasmine
For peace and comfort	Neroli, Linden Blossom, Chamomile
For liveliness and fun	Marjoram, Rosemary, Tuberose
For opening to universal abundance	Rose Otto, Neroli, Tangerine, Lavender
For clearing negative habits and thought patterns	Frankincense, Sandalwood, Carnation, Tuberose
For increasing confidence and self-worth	Geranium, Rose Maroc, Ylang Ylang
For connecting with your higher self	Rose Maroc, Jasmine, Neroli, Myrrh

CRÈME DE LA CRÈME

Leslie's favourite recipe for a sensuous and dreamy room spray. It's delicious, but not *cheap* to make:

- Rose   10 drops
- Jasmine   6 drops
- Linden Blossom 4 drops

Add the drops to a pint of water, add a drop of washing-up liquid, pour into your plant sprayer and shake well.

CALL TO ACTION

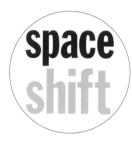

Set a Space-Clearing Date: Is your priority to clear a single room, an office, your entire home? Decide what space you want to address and choose a time you'll go for it. If you're having trouble sleeping, for instance, begin by clearing and dedicating your bedroom.

Collect Your Tools: Go through the Tool Kit list on p.165 and make a note of anything you might need. Make, borrow or buy the items on your list.

Scent Your Atmosphere: Even if you don't have time for a complete space-clearing ritual, treat yourself to the delight of a homemade room spray. Find single essential oils that you love, or blends, and make up your own bottles of blessing water (see p.166). Use the spray frequently to revitalize your home, car or workspace.

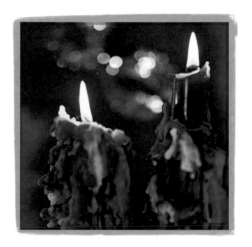

'Rituals and symbols can provide
the structure by which life experiences
yield new meaning.'
Carl A. Hammerschlag

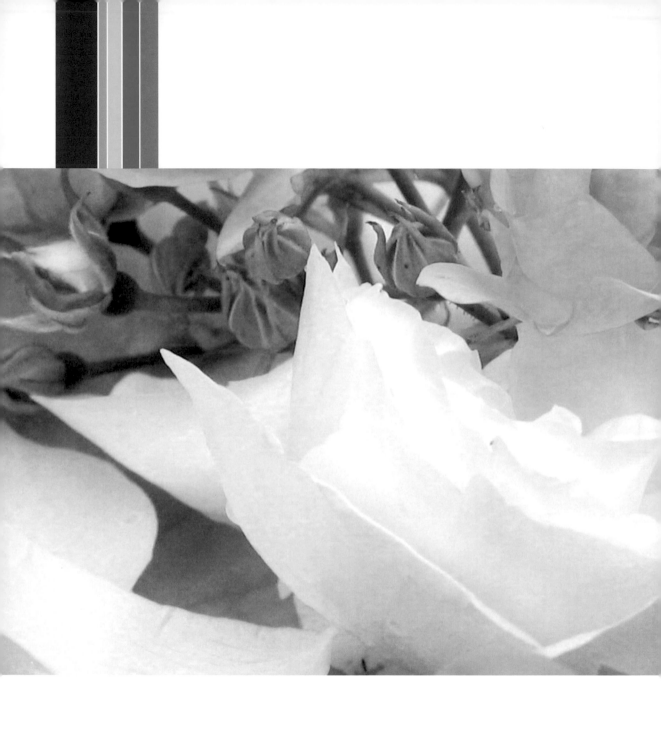

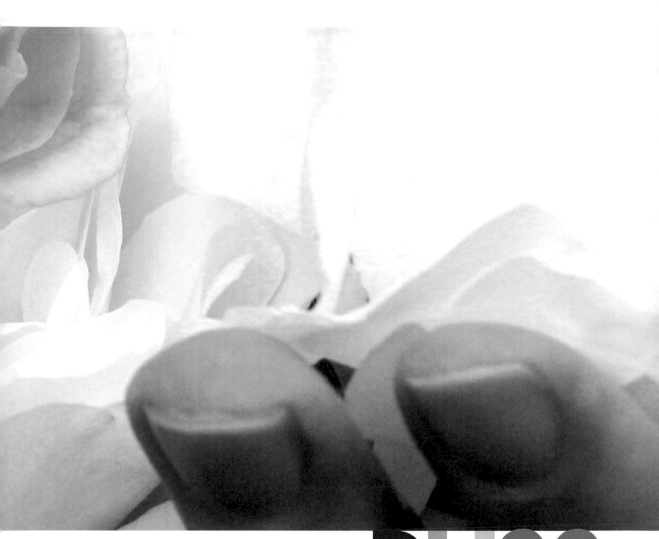

BLISS

12 DIVE INTO BLISS
embody ecstasy

'Follow your bliss', the gypsy said. 'Connect with your inner light. Hear the sounds of birds. Taste the ocean's spray. Listen to the whispers of your soul. You were born to it. Bliss is your key to freedom. Have you forgotten?'

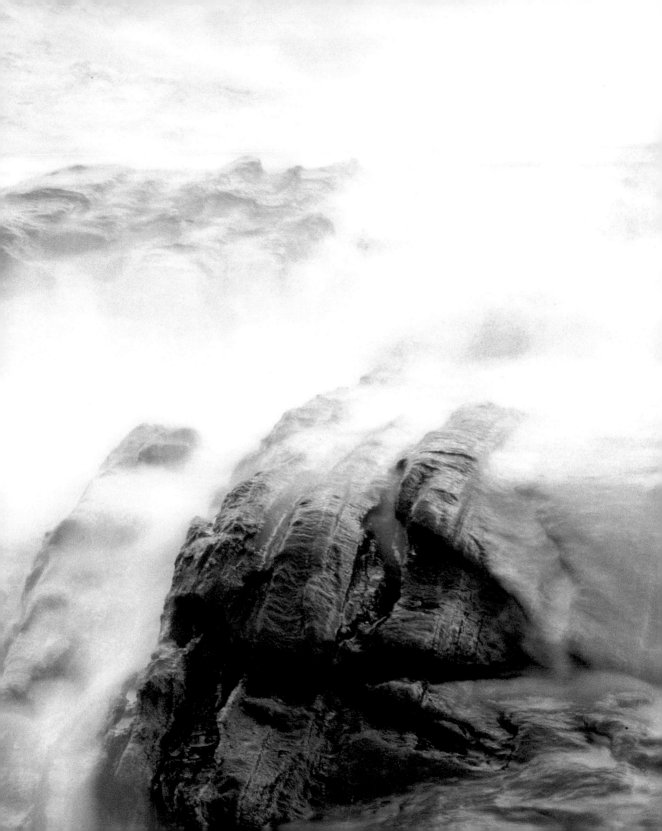

The gypsy's words echoed in the woman's heart. She had never followed her bliss. She had always tried her best to do the 'right' thing, listened to the voices of others and valued their opinions above her own. She'd been on and off slimming regimes, lost weight, gained weight, made money, spent money, found lovers, lost lovers, done assertiveness workshops and given up doing them. Occasionally she figured she'd found an answer to something. Then it would melt away again like some forgotten dream.

That was when she met the gypsy on the road. The gypsy was old and wrinkled. Yet her eyes shone with a light so bright the woman could hardly bear to look into them. 'What the hell', the woman thought, 'let's see what this old lady has to say. What have I got to lose?' That was the day the woman let bliss into her life – the beginning of a journey that would transform her body and illuminate her life.

'When I look into the future it's so bright it burns my eyes.'
Oprah Winfrey

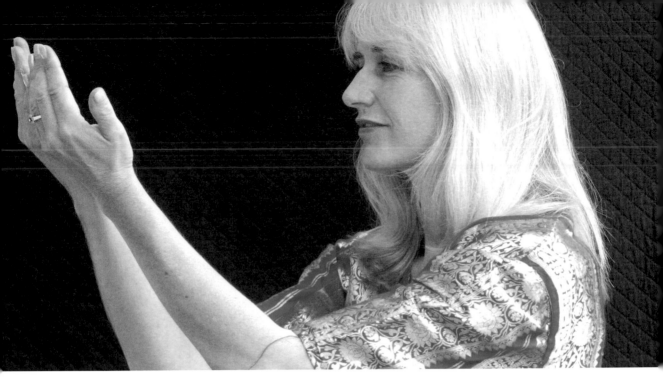

Follow Your Bliss

You can waste a lot of time and energy doing what you think you *should*. Living this way is a recipe for moving further and further away from soul connection and bliss. Instead, begin to explore what you *love*. When looking for the meaning of his existence Jung asked himself the question: 'What did I most love doing as a child?' He remembered he adored making little streets and houses out of stones and blocks. So he bought some land at the side of the lake in Zurich, and began to build a house with a tower. There was no rational sense to what he was doing. He already owned a fine house. But what he created for himself, in choosing to do this, was a sacred space within which he could both come in touch with and live out his deepest longings and fascinations. Honouring the whispers of his soul, Jung not only expanded his capacity for bliss. He set the stage for the finest writings he would produce during his life and embarked on a road to fulfilment he could not have imagined possible before. What do *you* love?

WIRED FOR IT

Long before you were born you were *wired* for bliss. You still are: its oceanic quality brings an experience of oneness and harmony. You first experienced it floating in the womb: relaxation, aliveness, security and the sense that life has purpose. All is right with the world. If you want to live in the fullness of your being and to connect with your creativity, vitality, radiance and beauty, invite more bliss into your life.

BLISS

In ancient India they had a name for it – *Satchidananda*. **This composite Sanskrit word is made up of three roots:** *Sat* **means being or existence.** *Chit* **translates as** *awareness* **or** *consciousness. Ananda* **means** *bliss.* **Together they describe a radiant, boundless state of being that carries a sense of infinite awareness and joy. Satchidananda brings the capacity to create worlds and forms out of itself. There was a time when such experience was reserved for saints and shamans. No longer.**

The capacity for bliss, as well as our need to experience it, is inscribed on the primitive brain – almost as deeply as our need for air, water and food. Bliss is the medium through which mind, spirit and emotions weave a tapestry of meaning. Bliss renews. Bliss cleanses. It makes us feel whole, solid, stable and alive. When we encounter something new, bliss tells us 'This is something I want to try.' Then it brings us the courage to go for it.

So important is bliss to becoming who you really are and realizing your goals – whether they be a strong, lean, beautiful body, a rewarding career or a dynamic empowering relationship – that when we deny our need for it, or forget how to experience bliss, we are forced to look for artificial substitutes. Addictions arise: to food, drugs, alcohol, sex – even ambition. Then these addictions disempower us, taking us further and further from the authentic freedom and satisfaction we long for.

Sometimes we steel ourselves against bliss out of guilt or misguided self-denial. Then we become as mechanical as the sharp-nosed spinster – nit-picking and critical of everything and everyone, most of all ourselves. Is bliss the be-all and end-all of life? Nope. Is it an essential ingredient in realizing your potentials on every level? You bet.

'The privilege of a lifetime is being who you are.'

Joseph Campbell

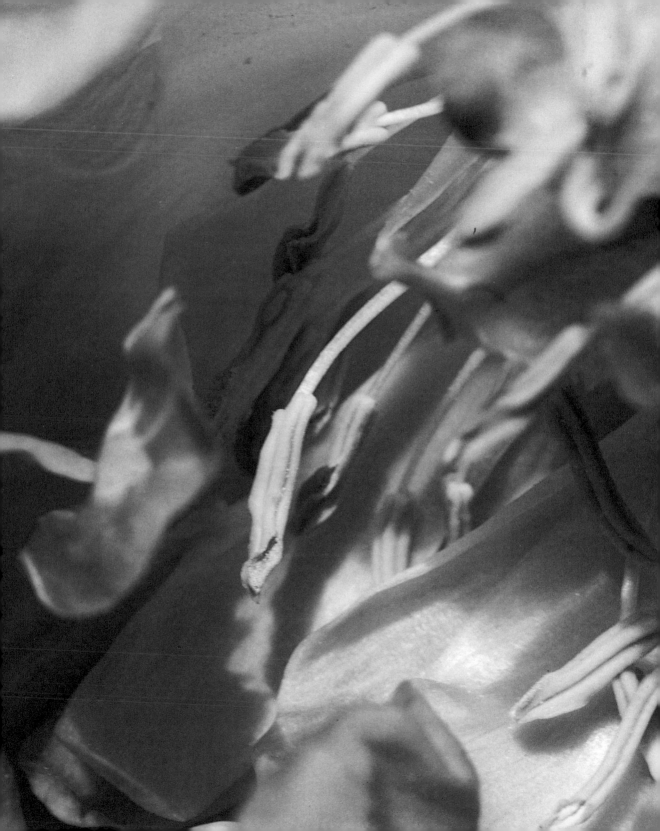

AWAKEN YOUR SENSES

All life is lived through your senses. The more awake they are, the more you will get out of the multidimensional pleasures of every moment: the aroma of freshly made coffee, the touch of silk against your breast, soulful fingers on guitar strings, waves of orgasm that swell your body and silence your mind. Forget everything you have been told about guilt and forbidden fruits: the secret to using bliss for transformation lies in becoming fully aware of everything you feel, touch, taste, smell, hear and see. Right here. Right now.

SCIENCE OF THE SENSUOUS

In the past 40 years scientists have begun to identify some of the biological carriers of bliss in our body. Pioneering research by Candice Pert at Johns Hopkins University, famous for her discovery of the brain's 'opiate receptors', and the work of others such as Avram Goldstein at Stanford and Lars Terenious in Sweden, have put bliss firmly on the map.

To put it in scientific terms, some kinds of bliss can be measured chemically. Peptides – endorphins and encephalins – connect with opiate receptors in every cell to create deep pleasure, relaxation and renewal. These peptides are part of the recently identified, infinitely complex tapestry of biochemistry, physicality and pure energy known as the living matrix.

'Molecules do not have to touch each other to interact. Energy can flow through... the electromagnetic field... The electromagnetic field along with water forms the matrix of life.'

Albert Szent-Gyorgyi

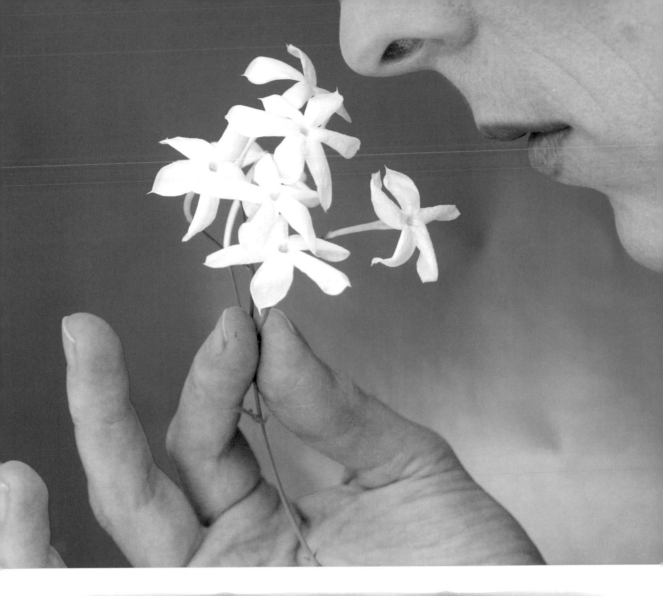

ENTER THE MATRIX

A high-speed communications system that involves all the systems in your body, the *living matrix* describes the rich tapestry of life that *is* you. When your matrix functions in harmony you experience radiant health, glowing skin and vitality no matter what your age. This living tapestry encompasses not only your organs and muscles, bones and sinews, but the electromagnetic field and energy grids that permeate your physical body and extend beyond it. The living matrix is the medium through which you experience bliss.

Imbibing Bliss

Some readers of our books are dying to know whether we 'survive' on a strict 'health-food' diet, or if we sometimes 'cheat'. If cheating means enjoying dark chocolate mousse, a frothy cappuccino or a glass of good red wine, the answer is most certainly 'Yes!' Except we don't consider it cheating. Our motto is, if you're going to eat chocolate, drink coffee or enjoy a bottle of wine, make it the very best. Savour it with every fibre of your being and above all don't ruin the experience by feeling guilty. Imbibe bliss with unadulterated hedonism.

CHOCOLATE THERAPY

Buy yourself a bar of rich, dark, organic chocolate. Unwrap the bar and break off a chunk. Smell the chocolate and anticipate the flavour. Put a piece in your mouth. Let it melt as you savour the texture and bitter-sweetness. Notice your thoughts. Are you able to stay in the bliss of the moment? Or is your mind filled with chatter? Can you activate your senses and simply drink in the pleasure of the moment?

GET REAL ABOUT CHOCOLATE

There are all sorts of imitation chocolates on the market with vegetable fat and lots of other junk added to them. Avoid them. Most chocolate is processed in an alkali medium. This makes it high in sodium and interferes with the absorption of the magnesium, copper, potassium, phosphorus, iron and calcium that pure cocoa contains. When buying chocolate, go for plain, bitter, dark chocolate, and choose organic. Not only is it the best, it's the most delicious.

'Some consider carob an adequate substitute for chocolate because it has some similar nutrients (calcium, phosphorus), and because it can, when combined with vegetable fat and sugar, be made to approximate the colour and consistency of chocolate. Of course, the same arguments can be made as persuasively in favour of dirt.'

Sandra Boynton – *Chocolate: The Consuming Passion*

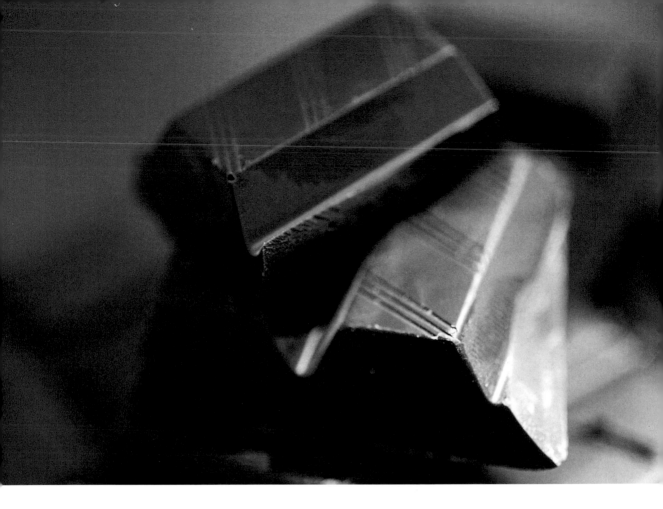

SACRED AND SEXY

Chocolate has long been considered sacred, with irresistible psycho-sexual properties unparalleled among foods:

- The Aztecs and Toltecs called chocolate the food of the gods. They told the story of how Quetzalcoatl, the supreme god of the air, brought the seeds of the tree to earth as a gift to his chosen people.

- Legend has it that Montezuma the great Aztec king downed 50 pitchers of an elixir made from chocolate each day. The drink, called xocolatl, was considered an aphrodisiac and fountain of strength, sexuality and vigour.

- When Cortez brought chocolate back to Europe in the 16th century, he created a chocolate storm among courtiers. Madame Pompadour gave her seal of approval to this black magic as an aphrodisiac. Casanova claimed chocolate was the perfect tool for seduction.

- Scientists have isolated a substance in chocolate which links into our brain's opiate receptors, which is why it brings sensations of pleasure and relaxation.

A Cup of Heaven

Another 'forbidden pleasure' is coffee. Like any food with alkaline drug-like properties and strong effects, coffee has been banned for periods throughout history. In the 16th century it was even forbidden in Mecca. But the Sultan himself so loved the beverage that he insisted it be made legal again. In the 17th century, the Catholic church did its best to ban coffee in Europe. Thankfully the Pope, an avid coffee drinker, opposed the ban. Soon afterwards coffee houses began to appear in both France and the United States, in the same spirit in which they exist today. They were places where people could meet, share a cup, and talk in an atmosphere of warmth and camaraderie.

'...coffee is bitter – a flavour from the forbidden and dangerous realm'.

Diane Ackermann – *A Natural History Of The Senses*

We love the spirit of coffee and the communal feeling it fosters. We consider the ritual of a good cappuccino enjoyed in excellent company one of life's great blessings. However, when we drink coffee, we are pretty choosy.

PERFECT BREW

Here's how we like it:

- **Organic**   Ordinary coffee is the most highly sprayed commodity in the world. Herbicides and pesticides can build up in the body to interfere with metabolic processes. Organic coffee is healthier and tastes better.

- Shade Grown   Unless coffee has been shade grown it is often cultivated by destroying valuable rainforests. Shade-grown coffee crops are planted beneath the rainforest canopy – helping us enjoy both the coffee and the rainforests.

- Fair Trade   This means that the workers who cultivate the coffee beans have not been financially exploited. Knowing that also makes coffee taste better.

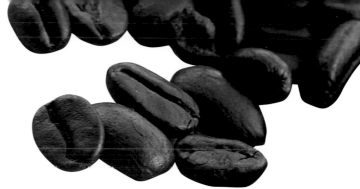

CAPPUCCINO À LA KENTON

We make our organic cappuccinos in large cups with plenty of frothy milk (organic cow's milk or soy milk). We use mostly decaffeinated coffee, with about 1/4 caffeinated for flavour and oomph. To the frothed milk we add 1/4 tsp powdered Coral Minerals (taken from land-based areas of Okinawa – see Resources). This does not affect the taste of the coffee, but has an alkalinizing effect to offset coffee's acidity. Lastly, we sprinkle the foam with cinnamon – which naturally supports blood-sugar balance – and with unsweetened organic cocoa. Then we drink our brew spiked with a dose of highly trivial conversation. A perfect blend.

GET WISE ABOUT COFFEE

Research shows that women who drink a lot of coffee while eating a high-fat diet have a greater risk of both breast cancer and bladder cancer. Similarly, drinking coffee during pregnancy increases the rate of birth defects and miscarriages. Even moderate coffee drinking can raise cholesterol levels in some. From the point of view of digestion, coffee can interfere with the assimilation of nutrients – one of the reasons why heavy coffee drinkers tend to be deficient in minerals. So if you choose to drink it, make it a pleasure not an addiction.

THE GOOD STUFF

Despite all the warnings, coffee can also benefit mind and body. Coffee warms, stimulates and has a natural diuretic and purgative effect on the body. The cafés in Paris in the last century were filled with famous writers, artists, politicians and thinkers, who enjoyed the stimulation that coffee (and good company) can bring.

RED, RED WINE

From years spent in France, we subscribe to the maxim that a glass of good red wine helps to relax the liver and fortify the blood. Red wine is considered superior to white because it contains higher quantities of health-boosting phytonutrients. We prefer our wine in large glasses that allow us to savour the aroma as well as the flavour. To enhance the bliss of the experience, we light a log fire, caress a cat and talk about love.

Total Immersion

An easy and accessible way to slip into bliss is getting into warm water. Set aside 20 to 30 minutes every so often to indulge your senses in a languid aromatherapy bath. Light candles. Play your favourite music. Lace the bath water with essential oils and immerse yourself. Close your eyes. Breathe in the mind-altering aroma. Allow your body to melt from a solid into a liquid state. Let yourself merge with the element of water. Water by its very nature is sensuous, renewing, healing. It is the stuff of baptism, blessings and regeneration.

'If there is magic on this planet, it is contained in water... its substance reaches everywhere; it touches the past and prepares for the future.'

Loren Eisley

AROMATHERAPY ALCHEMY

Plants capture the sun's photo-electromagnetic energies, and pass their blessings on to us in the form of essential oils. We not only benefit from inhaling the fragrances of these volatile and complex hydrocarbons, we take their tiny molecules in through our skin when we bathe in them. And our own energy fields are enhanced by theirs. This can bring about beneficial shifts in hormone levels, alter circulation and even change our breathing patterns. The tiniest amounts of essential oils can induce feelings of euphoria, heighten sexual desire, increase mental clarity or clear the negative effects of stress. Each essential oil has unique properties. Get to know them individually and you'll discover what good friends they can be in so many areas of your life.

Some essential oils stimulate. Others sedate. For a relaxing bath, choose an oil like lavender, whose action is sedative, and climb into warm rather than hot water: somewhere between 28 and 35°C. If you need invigoration, go for a stimulating oil, like neroli, and take a shorter, hotter bath: 35 to 39°C.

The simplest way to add aromatherapy to the bath is to sprinkle a few drops of essential oil into the tub once it's filled, swish the water around so that the oil droplets are well dispersed, then immerse yourself. Begin with 2 – 4 drops of essential oil per bath and gradually increase to 4-8 drops as your skin becomes accustomed to them (see Resources).

HOMEMADE BATH OIL

To moisturize your skin as you bathe, make your own bath oil blend. To each 1 – 2 teaspoons of avocado oil or sweet almond oil, add 1 drop of a mild shampoo and 2 – 5 drops of your choice of essential oils. Shake the mixture in a small glass jar and add a little to your bath.

Here are some of our favourite essential oils for bathing. Try them singly or in combination:

ESSENTIAL OILS FOR BATHS

To ease anxiety	Basil, Jasmine, Chamomile, Marjoram, Neroli, Ylang Ylang
To relieve depression	Clary Sage, Jasmine, Neroli, Rose Maroc
To soothe irritability	Marjoram, Chamomile, Lavender, Geranium
To diffuse anger	Ylang Ylang, Rose Otto, Chamomile
To strengthen body and mind	Helichrysum, Linden Blossom, Marjoram, Chamomile Maroc
To relieve stress	Rose Maroc, Chamomile, Lavender, Linden Blossom
To revive your spirits	Rosemary, Basil, Neroli
To wind down	Jasmine, Ylang Ylang, Lavender, Clary Sage, Melissa
To intensify sexual desire	Ylang Ylang, Patchouli

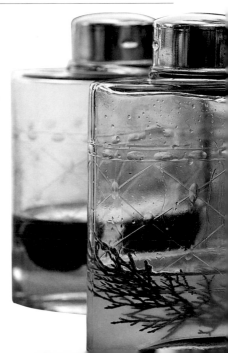

Breathe It

How you breathe affects not only how you feel about yourself but how much joy you experience. Shallow, upper-chest breathing can stress you out. It stimulates the 'fight or flight' response of the sympathetic nervous system. This is 'normal' breathing for many of us. Full abdominal breathing, on the other hand, helps you feel in control and at peace by bringing the restorative qualities of the parasympathetic nervous system into play. Practise the following exercise until it becomes second nature.

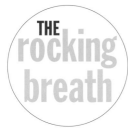

THE rocking breath

Lie on your back with knees bent, hands resting on your abdomen and soles of your feet to the floor. Sigh out, letting your muscles relax and melt into the floor. Begin slowly and gently to rock your pelvis back and forth, first pressing your tailbone into the floor while you arch your back and then tucking your tailbone under so that the small of your back flattens onto the floor.

Create a cycle of this pelvic movement switching gently from one position to the other about every four seconds. Notice how your breath begins to coordinate with the movement of your pelvis quite naturally: *As your tailbone tucks under, you exhale. As your tailbone rocks back and presses into the floor, you breathe in.* Notice too how your tummy gently rises with each in-breath and falls with each out-breath.

Continue this movement with as little effort as possible, allowing the rocking of the pelvis to refine itself until it feels completely natural – as if the breath itself is creating the movement. Once you get the hang of the pelvic movement, try it sitting or standing or even when making love. It can help you to tap into more and more of your innate capacity for bliss whenever you choose.

Towards the Vast Beyond

Heightening the bliss experience in day-to-day life begins in simple ways. Ask yourself a few questions about what brings you a sense of bliss, passion or enthusiasm in your own life. Working with your answers to these questions can help clarify who you are, what you value and what choices best serve the unfolding of your own beauty and freedom.

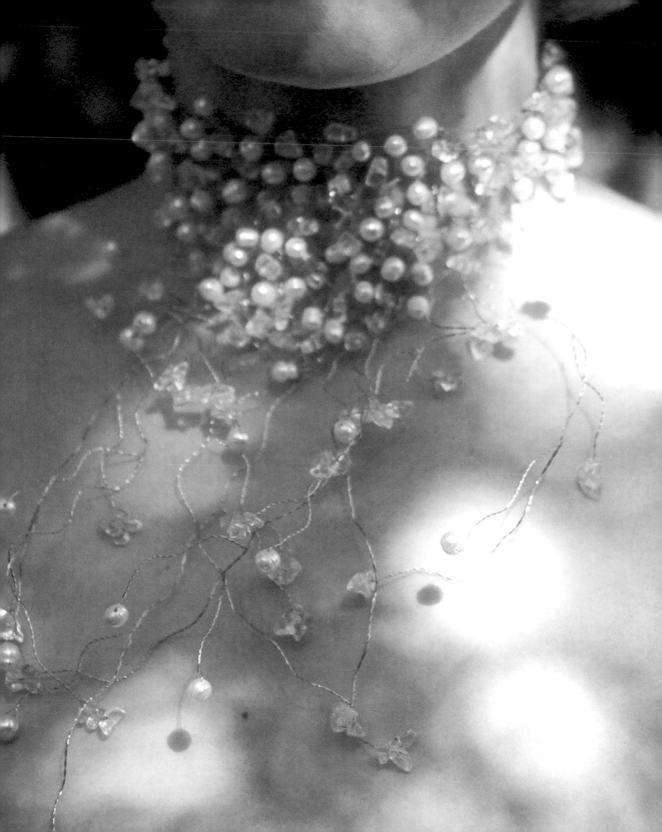

CALL TO ACTION

Prepare Your Authentic Path: Take out your Journal and answer these questions:

- What is the moving power behind my life today - what matters most to me?
- What did I love most as a child?
- How can I begin to live what I love most right now?

Explore these questions in an on-going way. It is the perfect antidote to the sense of meaninglessness that comes from following the wrong directives in your life – usually someone else's rules. Come back to what you've written whenever you feel you've lost your direction or purpose. Add to it as you hear more whispers from your soul. This can put you on the fast track to joy, freedom and authentic living.

Follow Your Bliss: Make time for an essential oil bath, a cappuccino with friends, and the very, very best chocolate you can find. Savour every second of it.

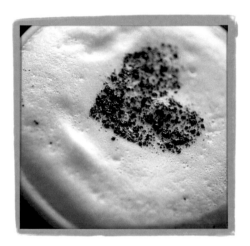

'The body feels the things of our
spirits that the mind never thought of.'
Carl A. Hammerschlag

13 SKIN GLOW
get real and look great

Your skin is *alive* – all twenty-one square feet of it. When you treat it as an inert surface to smear cream on, botox or put under the knife, it never realizes its full potential for bliss. Get savvy about what skin loves and hates. Then you can enjoy the rewards of firm, smooth, even-toned, glowing skin – naked or 'dressed' – at *every* age.

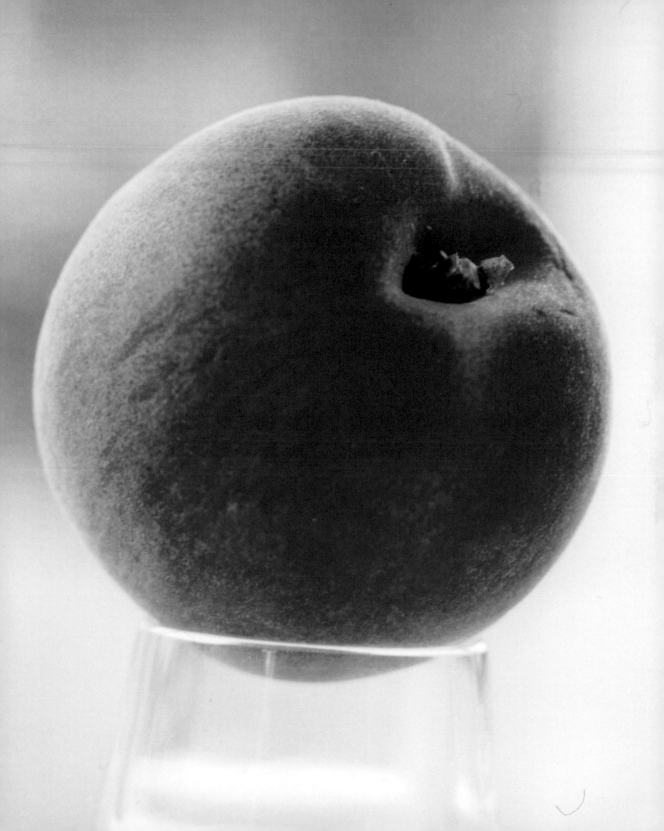

A multi-dimensional interactive system of information, molecules, energy, cells and genetic messages, skin is the living interface between you and the outer world. Its health and beauty is entirely dependent on the state of your living matrix. What you do *not* put on your skin – and into your body – is as important as what you do. Get the balance right and your skin will reward you with a glow that cannot be faked. Then if you decide to opt for surgery, botox or any other treatment, go for it. Here's the irony: once your skin becomes naturally radiant, such interventions can lose their appeal. There's a lot of fun that comes from looking great just as you are.

We stand at the brink of a revolution in beauty. Long awaited, its powerful ethos promises not only to transform your skin, it can even change your life. Rising from the ashes of fragmented thinking and commercial nonsense that has long dominated the cosmetics industry, the authentic approach to beauty and skincare carries power to transform the way you look and feel in ways never before possible.

Skincare products and self-care treatments for the authentic woman need to fit with the kind of clothes she wears, and the high-tech devices she uses – from iPods to portable ionisers – the organic foods she eats and the rowing machines she works up a sweat on. Few skincare manufacturers have yet switched on to the needs of the authentic woman. But it is coming.

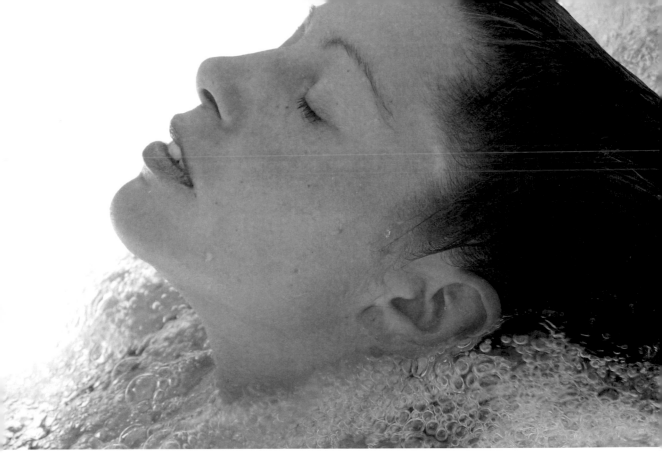

Clear Toxic Skin

When your blood is riddled with pollutants, your skin is starved of the nutrients it needs for healthy cell renewal. It ages quickly, sags and looks dull. Skin also becomes damaged through chemical and physical changes, some of which are irreversible. Clean up your blood and within days you can reawaken a youthful glow. That's how the Inner Face Lift Diet works its wonders. Try it (see p.38). Long term, protecting skin from toxic damage means understanding how widespread a threat this is and how to handle it.

Toxins that threaten the beauty of skin are everywhere – in the air we breathe, our food chain, the chemicals we clean our homes with and the majority of skincare products we use. The United Nations Environmental Programme calculates that 70,000 chemicals foreign to the human body are in common use across the world. Another 1,000 new chemicals get introduced each year, polluting the planet and our bodies. Legal loopholes in every country still allow beauty products to be sold containing potentially deadly toxins that disrupt the order of the living matrix, undermine skin beauty and provoke degeneration.

SKIN NEVER LIES

When your body is free of toxicity, when blood sugar and insulin levels are balanced, your skin glows. Fall in love and it radiates beauty. Plunge into depression and it responds by becoming slack, dull and lifeless. Skin gives an ever-changing, accurate measurement of your overall energy, vitality and emotions. Watch over it. Tend its needs with loving care and it will reward you.

CHEMICAL SEA

In the 21st century we live in a sea of toxic chemicals. Far more important than the potential harm any single chemical can do is the dangerous way in which these chemicals interact to produce even more compounds toxic to the body, with serious implications for skin beauty. It is not just the petrochemically derived oestrogen mimics carried in the air and sprayed on our foods, nor is it the chemicals in cleaning products, the artificial colourings and flavourings in convenience foods or even the phthalates and parabens in make-up and skincare products that are the problem. It's the build-up of all of these chemicals in our system, as well as even more toxic chemicals formed by interactions between them, that creates a *toxic load* in the body.

Your body can only handle so many chemical pollutants which, because they are foreign to living systems, are enormously difficult to shed. When the body's toxic load gets big enough, it becomes a toxic *overload*. This you want to avoid at all cost. Systems begin to break down, paving the way for wrinkled, sagging, lacklustre skin and degenerative diseases – from obesity and diabetes to heart conditions, PMS and menopausal disorders. Toxic load is increased by living on the standard Western diet, which fills your body with excess glucose, triggers Syndrome X (see p.80) and leads to early ageing and disease. The more toxic load you carry, the more your skin and body struggle to maintain health and good looks.

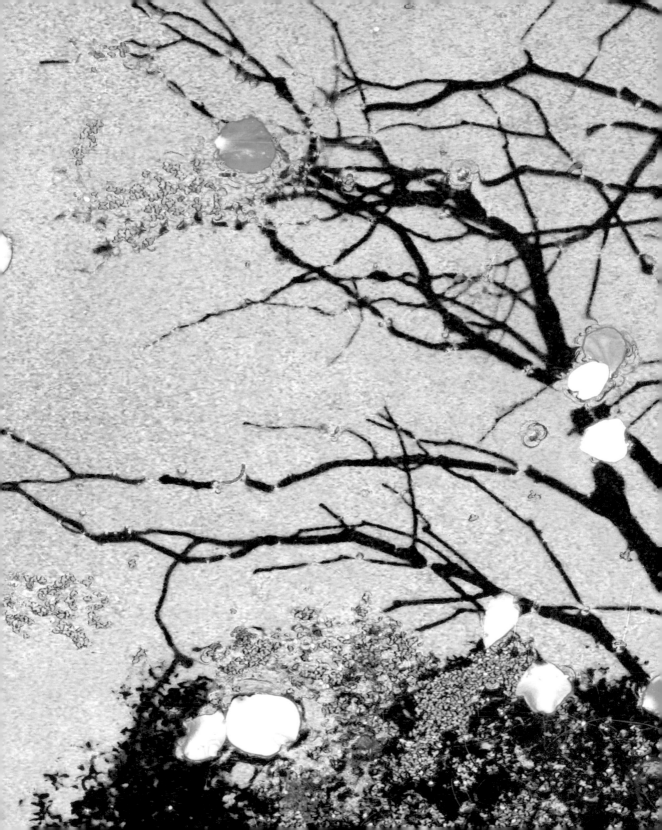

DUMP YOUR TOXIC LOAD

Decrease your toxic load to make skin more blissful.

- **Label Check:** Reduce your exposure to harmful chemicals by choosing your skincare and make-up products carefully. Cut back on use of products that contain any of the following (many of which are carcinogens): Parabens, DEA, MEA, TEA, Isopropyl Alcohol, Coal Tar Dyes, Artificial Fragrances.

- **Clean Sweep:** Clear your cupboards of household chemical cleaners, sprays and solvents. Opt for *truly* natural alternatives instead (see Resources).

- **Go Bio:** Eat organic foods rich in the minerals, vitamins and trace elements skin needs, and free from hormone-disrupting pesticides and herbicides.

- **Work It Out:** Get plenty of exercise. Walk for 30 minutes a day.

- **Breathe It Out:** Practise deep breathing to encourage the elimination of wastes through your lungs.

- **Smoke Free:** Stay away from cigarette smoke, both active and passive.

- **Clear Vibes:** Reduce your exposure to radiation from microwaves, computers, televisions and mobile phones, all of which disrupt the order of the living matrix.

- **Inner Wash:** Enhance elimination and kidney function by drinking at least eight 200ml glasses of purified/spring water a day.

- **Down Time:** Get plenty of sleep so your body self-cleanses and renews.

- **Sweat It Out:** Take a sauna often (our favourite kind is infrared – see Resources) to induce sweating, remove toxins and activate your skin's elimination processes.

'Beauty is but the spirit breaking through the skin.'

A. Rodin

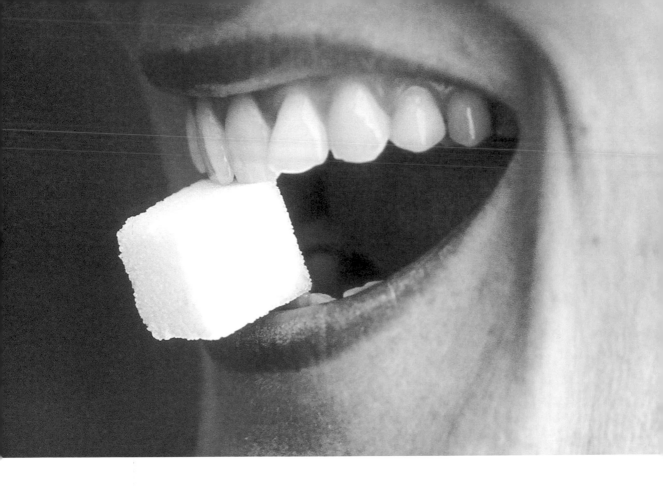

SWEET DEVASTATION

Kicking the sugar habit takes years off skin's biological age – firming sags, softening lines and increasing skin glow. *Sugar destroys skin.* Let's say that again: sugar destroys skin. Not just eating the white stuff, but pastries, pastas, breads and cereals – all of which turn into glucose and enter the bloodstream rapidly after digestion, causing the blood-sugar overload we talked about in Primal Food.

Where skin is concerned, the plot thickens. When glucose levels remain too high for too long, glucose binds to chains of proteins through an abnormal chemical process that resembles the charring of meat, to form *advanced glycosylation end products*, also known fittingly as AGEs. Skin functions become impaired, inflammation sets in, too many free-radicals are formed, sags and bags appear and your skin gets old fast. Excess glucose causes crosslinking, wrinkling and destruction to your skin's genetic material. As a result, cells reproduce abnormally, further undermining skin texture, tone and vitality. Radiance Eating halts rampant degeneration and turns all this sugar devastation around.

'Age is an issue of mind over matter. If you don't mind, it doesn't matter.'

Mark Twain

THE BEAUTY OF ORDER

Normal, healthy collagen and elastin form a network within the living matrix of skin. It looks a bit like beautiful hand-woven fabric with collagen forming most of the vertical weave. Collagen gives skin its structural integrity and density. AGEs cause collagen fibres to stick together and bunch up so they become rigid, losing their flexibility and strength. The first external signs of advanced glycosylation often show up as 'pillows' around the eyes. AGEs make your skin look soft and droopy. Cross-linking becomes apparent around the mouth too. Skin hardens and becomes less flexible. Eventually the cheek area is affected. Cross-linked collagen is a major reason for the deepening of the crease between the edge of the nose and the side of the lips – called the nasal-labial fold. In someone with advanced AGEs and cross-linking, the skin's surface becomes a map of lines, which form squares that grow deeper by the year the worse the cross-linking problem becomes.

EAT RAINBOWS

Your skin thrives on phytonutrients – the compounds in brightly coloured fruits and vegetables giving them their hues – many of which are antioxidants. They help protect it from age damage, calm inflammation, enhance its ability to hold moisture and improve its immune function. They also help counteract toxic load. Make a habit of drinking freshly made juices made from a variety of vibrant coloured vegetables like beetroot, spinach and carrots. When you shop for food, fill your trolley with the most colourful fruits and vegetables you can find – blueberries, plums, tomatoes, pumpkin, pink grapefruit, broccoli. Not only are they delicious, your skin will love you for it.

Keen to get on the Skin Glow fast track? Check out three little-known nutraceuticals which can radically transform the way your skin functions, looks and feels. We swear by them.

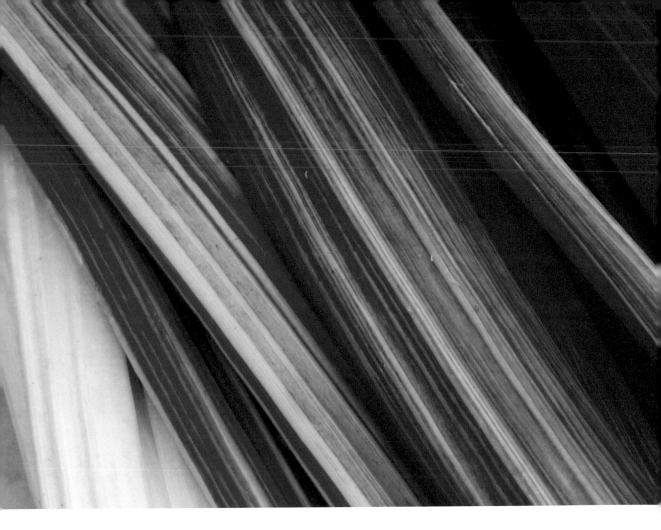

SMOOTHING SULPHUR

Sulphur is the hottest item in offices of savvy plastic surgeons these days, but it's a unique form of methyl-sulphonyl-methane, or MSM, that you want to use. MSM is found in every tissue of your body. Its concentrations diminish with age. Support your natural reserves by eating lots of fresh raw vegetables, fruits and seafoods – all rich in MSM. But, unless your diet is high-raw, it's unlikely you are getting enough for beautiful skin, let alone optimal health.

A good dose of MSM for beautiful skin is 2000 milligrammes (2 grammes) per day for each 60 kilos of your body weight. Start with 500 mg per 60 kilos of weight and work up. Always use MSM together with half the amount of vitamin C, preferably a buffered form such as calcium or magnesium ascorbate. (If you take 2g of MSM you would take 1 gramme of vitamin C.)

CONDITIONING CARNOSINE

The second master nutraceutical for skin is carnosine. Carnosine is a natural metabolite with powerful antioxidant properties found in particularly high concentration in long-lived cells like nerves and muscles. Concentrations in our muscles fall by more than 60 per cent between the ages of 10 and 70. Taking supplemental carnosine helps make up for this loss. This means firmer, more youthful skin. The recommended dose is 50 to 200mg of carnosine a day taken on an empty stomach.

RENEWING NICOTINAMIDE

A special form of vitamin B3, nicotinamide or niacinamide – the kind of vitamin B3 which does not cause flushing when you take it – has a stunning ability to reverse many aspects of skin ageing when used internally as a supplement and externally in skincare products. Nicotinamide:

- Increases collagen synthesis by stimulating the activity of fibroblasts.
- Decreases skin inflammation by inhibiting the release of histadine.
- Enhances the synthesis of lipids important for healthy cell walls and skin beauty.
- Diminishes wrinkles.
- Repairs DNA after skin has been exposed to too much UV light, electromagnetic or chemical pollution.
- Increases the biosynthesis of ceramides and other important moisture-holding gels in which skin cells are suspended.
- Fades age spots and helps prevent the formation of new ones.
- Plays a central role in blocking genetic messages which can result in skin cell ageing and death.

The usual dose of nicotinamide for improving skin is between 500mg and 1000mg a day. It is best taken with a good multiple B vitamin.

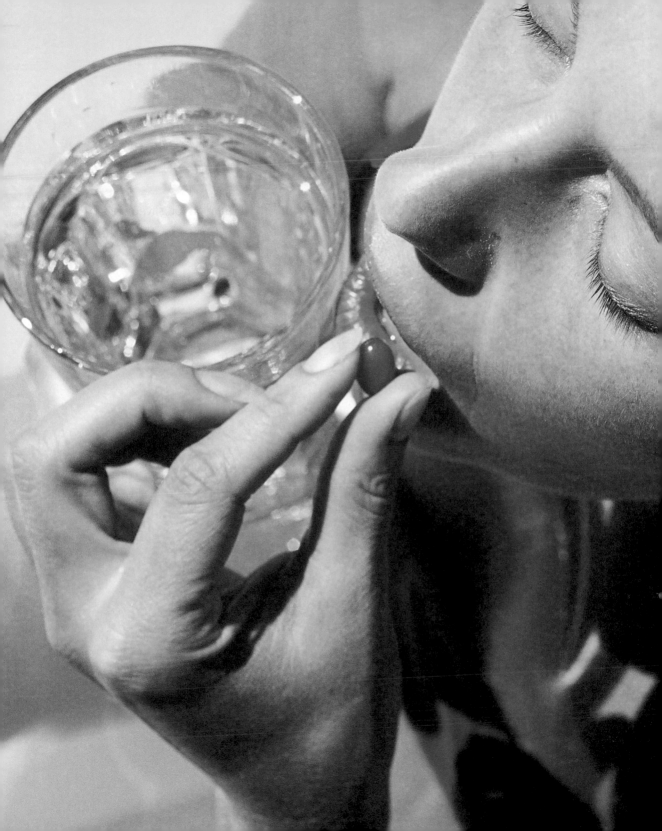

ELEMENTAL SUPPORT

A handful of other nutritional factors help round out an ideal formula for stunning skin. Like silica. This element has the ability to form lengthy complex molecules by binding with other elements. When it combines with magnesium and calcium, it creates firm bones, beautiful hair and nails and helps keep you free from cellulite. Fibroblasts need optimal quantities of silica as well as vitamin C, the bioflavonoids, copper and zinc to make good-quality new collagen. Research going back more than 20 years shows that getting enough of these elements helps prevent collagen breakdown and stabilizes the structures on which youthful and beautiful skin depend. Elemental support can undo much of the damage already done from neglect or poor nutrition.

LESLIE'S ELITE SKIN NUTRITIONALS

Here is our favourite regime for great skin. We use it daily as an addition to a top-quality multivitamin and mineral supplement including flavinoids, carotinoids and other plant factors (see Resources.)

- 3 g MSM
- 1500 mg Vitamin C
- 200 mg Carnosine on an empty stomach
- 1000 mg Nicotinamide
- 100-200 g alpha lipoic acid (ALA)
- 100 g Co Enzyme Q10
- 300 IU Vitamin E
- 100-200 mg Omega 3 Fish Oils containing DHA and EPA
- 1 tablespoon of Silica Gel

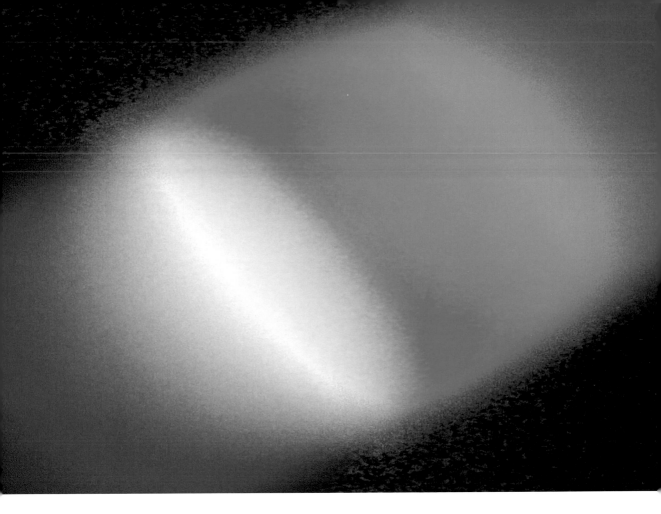

A Little Light Magic

New energy-based skin treatments and non-invasive technologies for professional skin treatments are being developed as we write. Take non-ablative skin rejuvenation – treatment that does not remove the surface of the skin. It uses intense pulsed light at specific frequencies to restore youthful feel and function to aged or neglected skin. Similar light-based treatments work other wonders: guided by the melanin (colour) in a person's skin, a few high-tech machines are capable of delivering a charge to hair follicles to disable growing hairs and allow unwanted ones to be shed permanently. This can be a godsend to women with 'moustache' problems and to men who since puberty have kept their shirts on at the beach, embarrassed about excessive hair on shoulders and back.

Then there is the exciting new grow-your-own-cell treatment. Known as Isologen, it may, before long, render injections of bovine collagen and silicon redundant. A person's own skin cells – fibroblasts – are harvested by a surgeon, cultured in a laboratory and later injected into areas of their face to clear lines, redefine smoothness, soften scars, and restore firmness and contours. Like dietary changes and some of the new biologically active skincare products, Isologen is a procedure designed to activate your body's own ability to create good-quality collagen.

HEALING LASER

The laser, another light-based treatment, which was once only used as an alternative to chemical skin peels, has been born again in a new form: called Low Level Laser Therapy (LLLT) it is a gentle, penetrating and healing form of coherent light, and an effective way of rejuvenating skin. Unlike most lasers, LLLT does not cut or burn. Instead, it enlivens and regenerates tissues through *photobiostimulation*, firming, revitalizing and encouraging the formation of new collagen. For many years this healing laser has been used with great success in the treatment of sports injuries, especially in Russia where light medicine and energy medicine are far in advance of Europe and the United States. Only recently has LLLT been applied to skin beauty. The results are excellent. Leslie was introduced to it by pioneering Russian doctor Lyudmila Nikolenko. Nikolenko combines 30 minutes of LLLT photostimulation with ten minutes of electro-acupuncture. Several treatments over a period of a few weeks brings such transformative results – smoother, firmer, more youthful and radiant skin – that plastic surgery can lose its appeal.

SUNLIGHT MATTERS

Your face, like the rest of your body, needs sunlight to look and function at its best. Biophoton research indicates that healthy skin cells 'suck order' from UV light and that this enhances the functioning of the living matrix. Skin behaves in a younger way and becomes more radiant. Get too much sun exposure and you can burn and damage your skin. Get too little and you miss out on the blessings the sun has to offer.

THE BRIGHT SIDE OF THE SUN

Exposure to sunlight:

- **Activates the production of ATP, raising cellular functioning to a higher level of vitality and creating a healthy glow.**
- **Increases the production of new collagen.**
- **Enhances the function of enzymes involved in cell repair and regeneration.**
- **Helps the lymph system clear wastes.**
- **Spurs the development of new capillaries.**
- **Enhances DNA functions and protein synthesis.**

SMART SUNBATHING

If you are unused to sun exposure, and especially if your skin is very fair, begin with short sessions of just 10 minutes and work up to half an hour a day. The best time to get in the sun is before 11am or after 3pm.

Women who conscientiously slather on sunscreen to protect themselves from skin cancer may inadvertently increase their risk of it. Sunscreens are made of chemicals absorbed into the skin that contribute to toxic overload and can be carcinogenic. It's far better to use hats and clothing to screen you from the sun, or to use products that contain inert substances like titanium dioxide and zinc oxide. Mineral make-up will protect your face.

Magical Mineral Make-up

Natural mineral-based cosmetics represent a unique technology in skincare, combining make-up, concealer and sun block all in one. They are made out of non-reactive elements like titanium dioxide and zinc oxide. Titanium is described by the American FDA as one of the purest and most effective ingredients available for sun protection. Zinc oxide has long been used to encourage the healing of skin disorders. Mineral foundations provide instant broad-spectrum (dealing with UVA, UVB and UVC rays), safe chemical-free *physical* protection from the elements. Unlike conventional foundations or sunscreens, they are not riddled with potentially harmful chemicals, dyes, preservatives, talc or perfumes to aggravate sensitive skin. And because their minerals are inert – in effect non-reactive – they don't support bacterial growth.

Mineral-based products are great, even for troubled skin, provided whatever you use to apply them is scrupulously clean. In fact mineral make-up is actually *good* for your skin. It is so calming that it can even be used after a skin peel. Little wonder cosmetic surgeons and dermatologists throughout the world are raving about it. Jane Iredale's mineral foundations – which we both use – carry an SPF between 17 and 20. One light brushing of foundation provides a sun block, which is both water- and perspiration-resistant, for day-long protection. You can even go swimming in it. Later it comes off easily with a cleanser.

LIP PRESS-UPS

We've become intrigued by a device known as a Facial Flex which fits in the corners of your mouth (making you look like a wide-mouthed frog). It allows you to exercise lots of the delicate muscles of your face isometrically without etching lines into your skin. Participants in clinical studies over an 8-week period, exercising just a few minutes daily with the instrument, showed an average 32.5 per cent increase in facial firmness (see Resources).

WISE CHOICES

If you've read all your skincare product labels in and discovered with horror that to be 'good' means parting with items you paid a small fortune for and love, take heart. There's nothing wrong with using a delicious face cream that contains a no-no, like parabens. But we encourage you to be conscious of the overall toxic load in your life and do whatever you can to *reduce it*. The next time you buy cosmetics, as a gift to your skin, use our guidelines in Resources.

LESLIE'S APPROACH TO BUYING PRODUCTS

I go out of my way to protect my skin and body from the build-up of chemical colorants, preservatives and sequestering agents which are ubiquitous in make-up and most toiletries. But I never make a 'religion' out of it. If I fall in love with a product – a lipstick, a mascara, or cream which *works* for me even though it contains something I would rather it didn't – I use it until I find something else that performs equally well and is purer.

EXTREME AUTHENTIC MAKEOVER

We're not opposed to cosmetic surgery and other beauty-enhancing procedures. At first glance it may seem there is something contradictory between *authentic* beauty and say, a rhinoplasty. We don't think so. If you feel that cosmetic dentistry, a face-lift or whatever, enables you to express who you are, we say go for it. Do it out of love for yourself, not from a place of self-loathing. Do it to express your uniqueness more fully. Let the procedure be an initiation into a more whole, fulfilled and happy you.

CALL TO ACTION

Toxic Dump: Begin to reduce your body's toxic load in simple ways: go for organic food, choose natural cleaning supplies, explore pure skincare products. Even small changes can have a big impact.

Skin Food: Increase your intake of colourful phytonutrient-rich fruits and vegetables to enhance your skin's radiance.

Elite Magic: Investigate some of Leslie's Elite Skin Nutritionals, including MSM, Carnosine and Nicotinamide, to see what they can do for your skin.

Finishing Touch: Protect and enhance your skin with a mineral foundation.

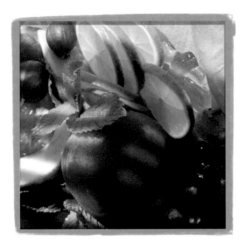

'Women who live for the next miracle
cream do not realize that beauty
comes from a secret happiness and
equilibrium within themselves.'
Sophia Loren

14 COME ALIVE
tune in and turn on

Your genes are encoded with the need to dance, to run, to dive into water and tingle with joy at just being alive. As kids, we know this instinctively. We moved for the fun of it. As adults we have forgotten how. We call movement 'exercise' and what was a joy becomes a duty – the biggest 'should' of them all.

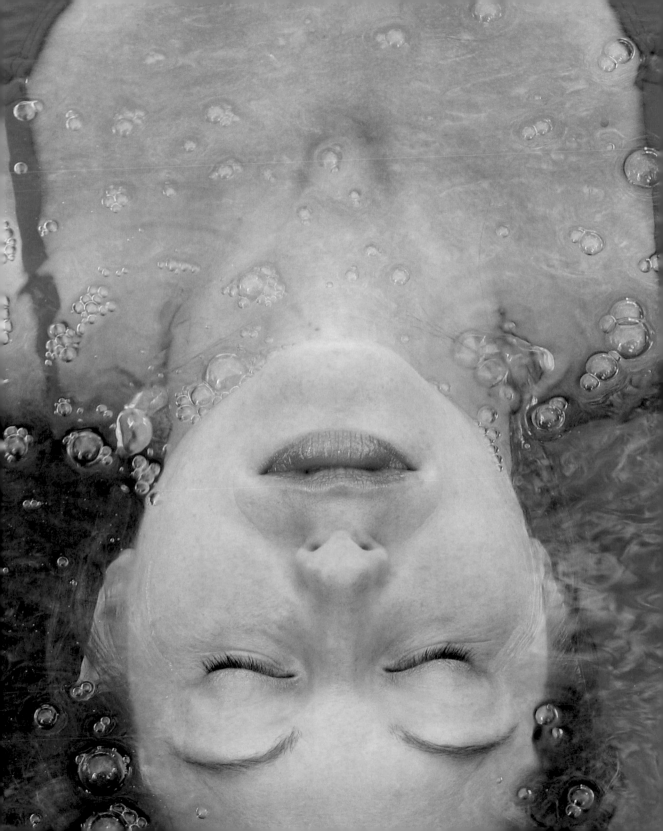

Forget about exercising to trim a thigh or protect your heart. Regular dynamic movement can do both, but the real payoffs are far greater. All our lives we are urged to do something for the sake of something else. Get a degree so you can get a job, so you can earn money, so you can buy what you want and so on ad nauseum. It's time to explore movement *for its own sake*. Your body and mind, feelings and senses wake up when you move. You think more clearly. Your self-esteem blossoms – you become fully alive.

A New Approach

Movement is a fundamental expression of your *embodiment* – how well your soul and your body are merged, in other words, how authentic you have become. Central to living in your truth and power, full embodiment is what can turn dreams into reality. When you exercise with the intention of honouring your body's need to move and open yourself to the pleasure of it, a shift takes place deep within the limbic system of your brain that dramatically alters how you perceive yourself and your life. It can clear a sense of impossibility and empower you to create the life you want.

> 'Most of us don't become what we can because we can't see it's what we already are.'
>
> **Carl A. Hammerschlag**

POWER CENTRE

The limbic system is a structure the size of a walnut embedded near the centre of your brain. A powerhouse of activity related to human emotion, behaviour and survival, your limbic system mediates passion, desire and drive. It is the filter through which you interpret experiences – good or bad. When it functions in a balanced way, your limbic system brings spice to your life, a positive outlook and hope. When it becomes inflamed or hyperactive you interpret even neutral events through a *negative* lens. 'Feeding' the limbic system with what your body craves – movement, touch, sound and pleasure – leads you to see life through a bright lens. And, because of how the limbic system influences motivation, nurturing its need for movement is also central to fulfilling your goals and realizing your dreams.

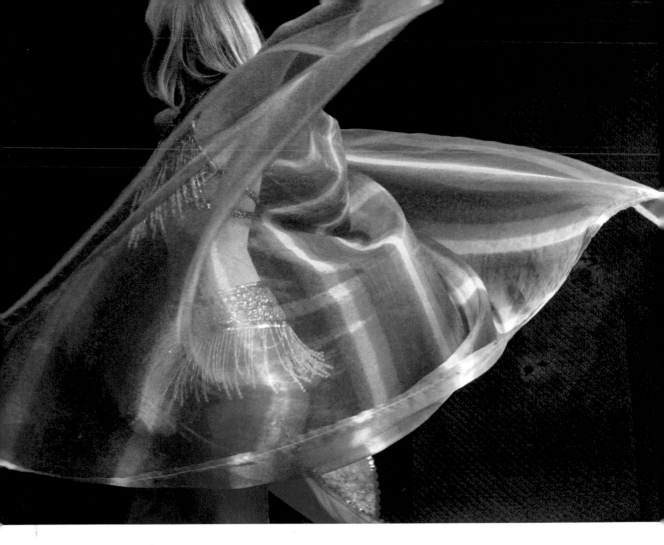

SEXUAL FEEDING

Like moving for the joy of it, healthy sexuality feeds the limbic system. It brings a sense of bonding and fulfilment. Random one-night stands, on the other hand, create disharmony in the limbics that can lead to dejection and despair. Sexual food for thought.

LIMBIC WORKOUT

American expert in limbic exercise, Majid Ali, M.D, describes two opposing approaches to working out. The first he calls *cortical exercise*. This is goal-driven, competitive and performed under the command of the thinking mind. It's the kind of exercise most people grit their teeth and bear. They decide on the amount of time they will exercise and the intensity they 'should' aim for, then go for external pay-offs. Such exercise, says Ali, depletes the body of energy (ATP) molecules while increasing levels of fatigue and stress chemicals. Cortical exercise has benefits, granted, but it does not shift consciousness, connect you with depths of transformative power, or restore your whole being.

Limbic exercise is non-goal-oriented and as such is an ideal way to move beyond the habit of using your will to flog your body into action. It allows you to explore, in an easy, natural way, the bliss of motion. Like other integral practices, it is movement for movement's sake, not something you do while you watch a TV monitor, plan the day ahead or hope to hell it will all end soon. Often carried out with eyes closed, limbic movement brings time for inner reflection, meditation, prayer and visceral awareness. It has the opposite physiological effects to cortical exercise. It reduces the number of fatigue molecules in your body, increases the number of energy molecules and leaves you feeling restored at the end of a workout instead of wiped out.

go limbic Choose an activity you can do with your eyes closed – maybe working out on a rowing machine, an elliptical trainer, a stationary bike, dancing, or simply jogging in place. Begin to move gently. Focus your gaze softly on an object ahead of you. Then allow your eyelids to become heavy and to close. As you move, become conscious of how your body feels – your muscles, your inner organs, your skin, your breath. 'Listen' to your body and let it move in whatever way *feels* best – sometimes fast, sometimes slow. Just follow its rhythms and enjoy. There is no set time limit for how long to continue. Your body will tell you when you are done.

'Music is the mediator between the spiritual and the sensual life.'
Ludwig van Beethoven

Your Resonant Body

A marriage of good music and movement can also create limbic bliss. Listening to music while you exercise is a great way to enjoy physical activity and end exercise drudgery.

The universal language, music bridges all cultures and continents because it affects the human body and spirit so deeply. For thousands of years it has been used for healing and regeneration. Like a piano or a guitar, your body is a resonator. When sound reaches it, the pulsations vibrate through your tissues. Sounds beneficial to you create greater order within the living matrix, producing an experience of pleasure and meaning. When listening to a violin concerto, for instance, the brain's electrical impulses shift into a relaxed alpha state. A fast tempo in a major key induces happiness. Stately music in a minor key calls forth rich emotions, while dissonance, à la Schoenberg or Heavy Metal can induce anxiety and fear, creating limbic stress and shifting perceptions of reality towards the negative.

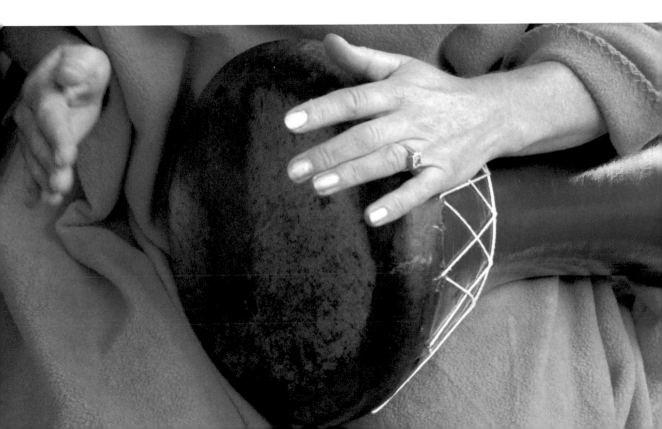

ENTRAIN YOUR BODY

Music intensifies the joy of movement because of the way it *entrains* body and mind. A physics phenomenon of resonance recognized for three centuries, entrainment is defined as the tendency of two oscillating entities to lock into phase so that they vibrate in harmony (in this case your body/psyche with the music you listen to). It was first identified in 1665 by Dutch scientist Christian Huygens. He discovered that when he put two pendulum clocks next to each other and set them running, before long they would mysteriously become synchronized – that is entrainment.

In the past 40 years a whole technology of entrainment using sound has developed to a high degree of sophistication. It involves the synchronization of brainwaves as well as different parts of the brain for the purpose of altering consciousness and supporting personal development. Making use of entrainment by bringing together music and movement is equally powerful for transmuting negativity, creating a high level of vitality, releasing stress and re-establishing harmony and serenity.

When the rhythms of a body in motion – whether it be walking, dancing, rowing, strength training or what-have-you – meet the complexity of ordered sound, all sorts of amazing things happen. Virtually every one of them – from balanced heart rate to stress reduction and a sense of pleasure – are mediated through the limbic system.

'Music expresses that which cannot be said and on which it is impossible to be silent.'

Victor Hugo

CHOOSE WITH PURPOSE

No question: music can also make you sick and sap energy. Think of the insipid stuff they play in supermarkets. A diet of depressing Country and Western laments floods the mind with negative thoughts – 'my man cheated on me, the money's gone, the dog's dead'. But classic Blues can transmute depression and despondency into resolution and peace. When choosing music to exercise with, be led by your instincts, not your logical mind. For example, don't automatically go for something peppy if you are feeling low. Try music sequencing: start with something in keeping with your mood, then gradually, perhaps, move to more upbeat tunes.

FEEL IT

While you exercise to music move your consciousness into your body. Sense the rhythm of your muscles as they contract and release. Feel the vibrations of the sound interacting with your body. You may even reach a point at which you and the sound become one. When the music stops and your movement ceases, listen to the silence. Feel the tingling stillness in body and mind.

THE TREASURE OF TECHNOLOGY

Use a personal stereo or better still get yourself an MP3 player. We both use iPods while we exercise. Start your own collection. Develop a wide range of music for working out. If you adore rock, great. Add it to your mix, but try other things too – Mozart when you want balancing, *Riverdance* when you want to soar, maybe Gorecki's *Symphony of Sorrowful Songs* when you need to release sadness. The possibilities are endless.

'Wagner's music is better than it sounds.'
Mark Twain

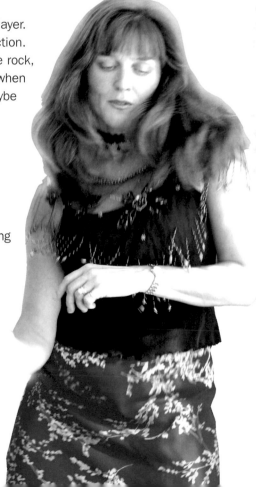

DANCE IT

Gabrielle Roth has some good music for movement including *Music for Slow Flow Yoga, Refuge* and *Tribe*. Her 'shamanic' *Five Rhythms: Flowing, Staccato, Chaos, Lyrical and Stillness* are good for entrainment, through dance. According to Roth, moving through these rhythms in order is like moving through the natural stages of life. Each one has its own qualities and rewards. The sequences shift consciousness and bring you to a place of emptiness where you *become* the dance. She describes her rhythms as 'markers on the way back to… a very vulnerable, wild, passionate, instinctive self.'

CALL TO ACTION

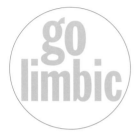

Limbic Spells Pleasure: Try the Go Limbic exercise. Notice how different this way of moving is from regular exercise. Are you able to tap into the bliss of motion? Make a note of any insights you get in your Journal.

Music Boost: Take time to create a collection of CDs, or to gather MP3 files to accompany your workouts. Choose pieces that inspire you and suit different moods.

Find Your Rhythm: Explore ecstatic dance *à la* Gabrielle Roth. You might like to take a class, if one is available in your area. Otherwise you can order her CD *Endless Wave Vol. 1* which talks you through the process of the five rhythms. Or discover your own rhythms by improvising to any music you choose.

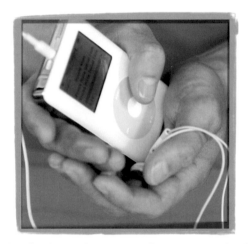

'Music has the capacity to touch the
innermost reaches of the soul and
music gives flight to the imagination.'
Plato

15 BODY BREAKTHROUGH
go wild and free

Dawn breaks. The woman slips from bed into her running gear. The house is still asleep as she creeps out the back door and pads softly along the pavement. Her lungs fill with the morning air and the scent of jasmine from a neighbour's garden. As her steps and breath join rhythm, she eases into *her* time — at peace, alive and free.

Once you rediscover the joy of movement for its own sake, your integral exercise practice, dedicated to fulfilling your core desires, can easily become the highlight of your day. To dissolve resistance and help you get moving, let's clear any nasty 'shoulds' you may have picked up from the media, health authorities and others.

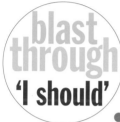

Take out your Journal and use it to complete the following sentence several times: 'I should exercise because…'

Example: I should exercise because:

- I need to burn off the calories from the tub of ice cream I ate yesterday.
- I'm embarrassed to be seen in a swimsuit looking like this.
- I've let myself go since my children were born.

Take a look at your list. How many of the reasons you wrote down are based on fear or self-judgement? Because they lack enthusiasm and passion, such reasons don't provide great incentive to get active.

Go for 'I Want'

Now repeat the same exercise, but this time complete the following phrase: 'I want to exercise because…'

Example: I want to exercise because:

- I love how my body and mind feel so alive after physical exertion and want to feel that often.
- I want to get fit enough to fulfil my dream to climb Mt. Kilimanjaro.
- I want to sculpt a lean, strong, beautiful body.

Movement Mantra

Look at your list. Notice how the reasons you've listed this time are more inspiring. That's because they are aligned with core values and desires. Choose the reason that has the most 'juice' for you. Write it out as a mantra. Put it in the present tense as if it already exists.

- I work out often and feel fully alive.
- I conquer Mt. Kilimanjaro feeling fit.
- I create a lean, strong, beautiful body.

Put your mantra where you'll see it each day – on your dressing table mirror maybe – to inspire your integral movement practice.

L.A. GYM STORY

'I once joined a gym in Los Angeles that offered members a free session with a personal trainer. At the beginning of my session the trainer asked me what my fitness goals were. "I'd like to become stronger," I told him. He nodded knowingly, "Yeah, what you want is a hard bod, firm tush, tight pecs..." I interrupted him, imagining I had not made myself clear, "Actually, I'm not really concerned with looking tight or hard, I'd just like to be stronger and to feel more alive in my body." "Oh right, like you don't wanna compete or anything, you just wanna look hot." ... I decided we'd settle for "hot".'

Susannah

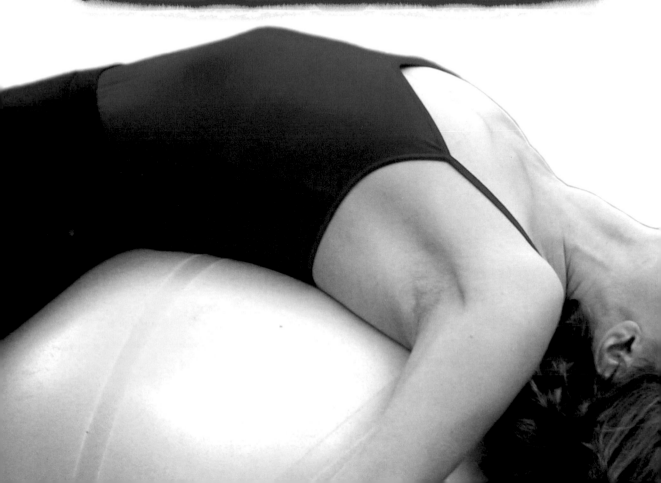

Dig Within For Bliss

Perhaps you've already discovered a form of exercise (or several) that you love. If not, this process helps you explore from the inside out activities that may make your heart sing.

Take out your Journal. Drift back to a time in your life when you were physically active and having fun. It may be from your childhood or teenage years, or it could be a more recent memory. Let the daydream evolve. Ask yourself what you enjoyed most about the activity, then write about it.

Example: Learning to tango. What did I enjoy most?
● Being transported by the music.
● The drama and self-expression.
● Dancing with a partner and communicating through the dance.
● The mental challenge of learning new steps.

Now use what you have written to identify your own personal keys to exercise fulfilment. Brainstorm about which activities might be most fun for you.

Example:
● Whatever workout I choose, even if it's just walking, I want to do it to music.
● I might take a dance class – salsa? swing? flamenco? – or study a martial art.
● I like working out with someone. Maybe I'll find a friend to take classes with.
● I might try the Brazilian Dance video I saw at the library.

Repeat the process using other memories of fun activities, such as in-line skating, volleyball, rock-climbing, horse riding, hiking.

You may find one form of movement you love most or come up with a kaleidoscope of activities which, together, sound fun. Once you have made a choice, schedule time for it in your calendar. To reap the greatest rewards from exercise for transformation, eventually you'll want to aim for at least 30 minutes of aerobic movement three to five times a week. It can be as simple as going for a walk.

Still need help choosing a form of exercise? Here are some suggestions and incentives:

WALK TO FREEDOM

Walking is an ideal integral practice. It is simple, can be done anywhere, any time, and leaves your mind free for contemplation. Walking at a brisk pace (15-minute mile or 4mph) brings most of the benefits of jogging over the same distance but without the same risks of injury or joint pain.

- **Deepen Your Practice:** Use your walk to expand consciousness with the Walking Meditation (see below).
- **Take a Friend:** Try walking with a two-legged or four-legged companion. Dogs have infinite enthusiasm for the 'w' word. It can be contagious.
- **Power Walk:** As you walk, become aware of your centre of power – a place a couple of inches below the navel. Imagine it moving powerfully through space, directing your arms and legs.
- **Vision Quest:** Use your daily walk to seek the solution to a challenge you face. Set the intention to receive guidance. Open your senses and take in 'messages' – a bird flying overhead, the pattern of bark on a tree, the colour of a car that passes you. Tune in and discover what the universe is telling you.
- **Extra Juice:** If you enjoy competition, why not consider training for an event, such as a walking marathon or charity walk?

'My grandmother started walking five miles a day when she was sixty. She's ninety-seven now, and we don't know where the hell she is.'

Ellen DeGeneres

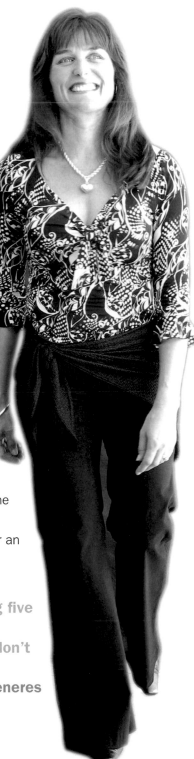

INSTANT RENEWAL

Dynamic exercise clears excess adrenaline build-up, renewing your sense of vigour and freshness. After a hard day, when you feel completely exhausted or irritable, resist the temptation to collapse on the sofa. Instead, move your body – dance, walk, swim, do Qi Gong. You'll be amazed to find that in about 30 minutes the energy you lost miraculously returns.

Walking Meditation

This is a fun meditation Susannah learned from teacher Byron Katie. It helps to still the mind and bring you into the present moment: begin to walk, and as you do start to notice and name what you see silently in your mind. Imagine you are God naming things for the first time. For example, you might see, and say: 'path...tree...bird...house'. When you feel your mind drift into other thoughts, such as what you are going to do later in the day or how you are feeling, simply bring your attention back again to notice what's around you and name it. Keep your mind on so-called 'first generation' thoughts. In other words 'leaf' not 'leaf on the tree that looks like it could use a good trim...' Notice how clear and centred you feel at the end of your walk.

MOVE FOR WELL-BEING

Regular, vigorous activity reduces anxiety and promotes long-term wellbeing, according to Tom Curetin at the University of Illinois. He studied 2,500 sedentary people who took up exercise. The result? Energy levels soared while tensions fell away. Similarly, Herbert de Vries at the University of Southern California looked at stress levels and muscle tension in subjects taking tranquillisers and compared them with those who engaged in daily physical activity. He found that exercise – even as little as a 15-minute walk – is more efficient in dealing with stress than a course of tranquillisers.

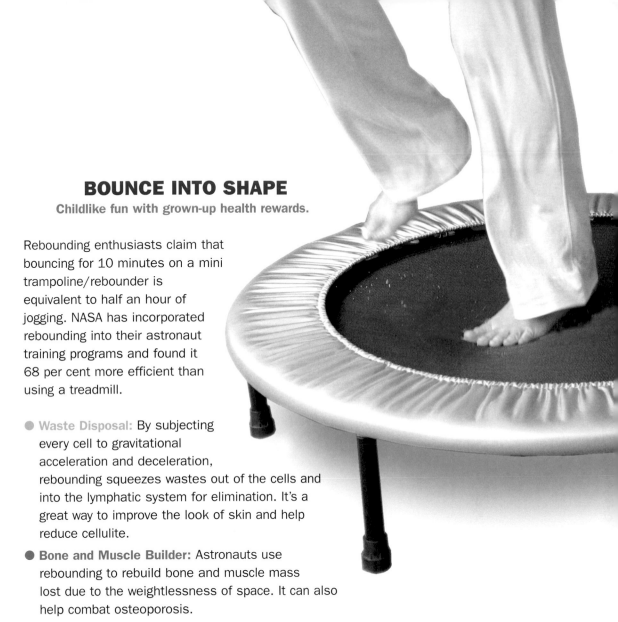

BOUNCE INTO SHAPE

Childlike fun with grown-up health rewards.

Rebounding enthusiasts claim that bouncing for 10 minutes on a mini trampoline/rebounder is equivalent to half an hour of jogging. NASA has incorporated rebounding into their astronaut training programs and found it 68 per cent more efficient than using a treadmill.

- **Waste Disposal:** By subjecting every cell to gravitational acceleration and deceleration, rebounding squeezes wastes out of the cells and into the lymphatic system for elimination. It's a great way to improve the look of skin and help reduce cellulite.

- **Bone and Muscle Builder:** Astronauts use rebounding to rebuild bone and muscle mass lost due to the weightlessness of space. It can also help combat osteoporosis.

- **Physical Rehab:** Rebounding helps athletes recover from injury. It's also ideal for the disabled, elderly and obese. (You can attach a frame to the rebounder to support balance.)

- **Spice It Up:** Listen to music/audio books as you bounce, or watch a favourite TV programme or film. Try a rebounding workout video for extra incentive. Add hand weights as you bounce to increase upper-body strength. Rebound indoors or outdoors.

'I think the key is for women not to set any limits.'
Martina Navratilova

SWIM IN BLISS

Merge with the medium of life.

Swimming helps develop long, beautiful muscles and firms skin. It is an ideal aerobic choice if excess weight or injury make it difficult for you to do weight-bearing workouts.

- **De-Stress:** Entering the medium of water itself is meditative. As you swim, let your breathing become rhythmic and let your stresses melt away.
- **Lower-Body Boost:** Use fins and a kickboard as part of your workout to target the muscles in your lower body.
- **Think Comfort:** Invest in a pair of goggles that don't leak and are comfortable. Kaiman goggles, made for triathletes, are especially good.
- **Get Organized:** Take the hassle out of trips to the pool by organizing a swimming kit with everything you need to get showered after your swim. You might include: a clarifying shampoo, a rich conditioner, a loofa, delicious-smelling shower gel, body lotion, moisturizer and a hair dryer.
- **Go Natural:** When you have the opportunity, swim in the ocean or in a lake instead of a swimming pool. There is nothing like the invigoration of a salt-water or fresh-water plunge.

MOOD MENDER

If you suffer from depression, look to exercise for relief. Psychiatrist John Greist conducted a study with depressed university students. He treated some with conventional psychotherapy and asked others to run for a few minutes each day. After ten weeks he reported that the runners felt better, studied better and did better in their exams than the conventionally treated group.

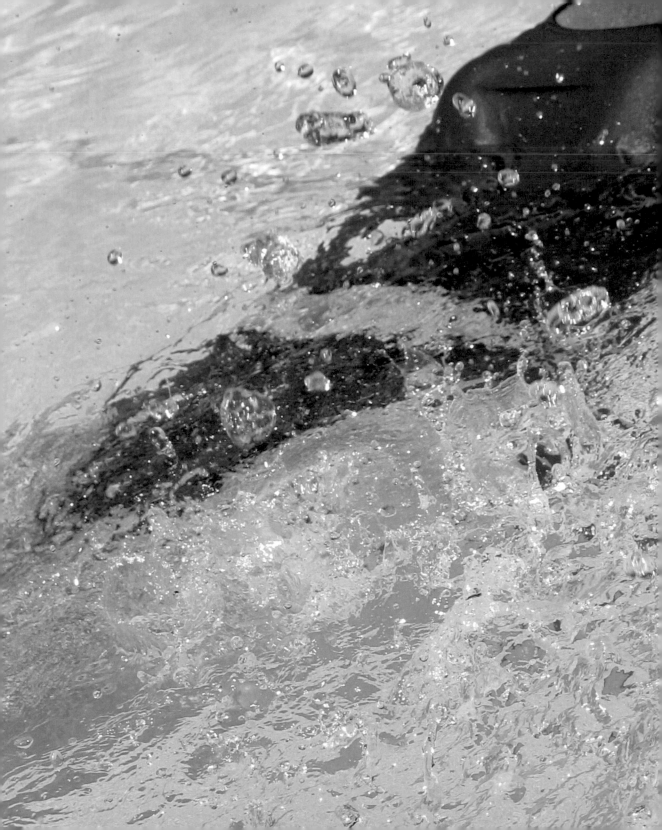

WORK OUT WITH THE BEST ON DVD

A smorgasbord of activities for your delight.

Turn your home into an inspiring exercise studio. Take classes with some of the world's finest teachers at the touch of a button with exercise DVDs, videos and CDs. Create your own library with selections to suit your every mood.

- **Feeling Aggresive?** Try a kickboxing DVD. Channelling anger into punching and kicking can be liberating, empowering and fun.
- **Want To Strengthen Your Core?** Look to Pilates. It not only improves posture and can alleviate back problems, it strengthens the important core muscles. Right in the centre of the body, around the navel, is the place where not only your physical power is centred, but also your sense of individual strength. Strengthen this area and the whole of your life becomes easier.
- **Feeling Disconnected?** Yoga is ideal for grounding and centring. A power yoga DVD can give you a great aerobic workout in addition to the benefits of stretching. A gentler one can help you de-stress.
- **Want To Sweat and Have Fun?** Try an aerobic dance DVD with an exhilarating beat to get you moving, such as African dance, salsa or even belly dancing.

EASY DOES IT

A motivational speaker we know once described how she began a fitness programme to lose 30 excess pounds. 'The first morning, I put on my running shoes and looked at myself in the mirror. Then I took them off. Day Two I put on my running shoes, shorts and a tee shirt and walked to the kitchen and back. The third day I got kitted up, stepped outside and took a few deep breaths...' As it happened, she eased into a regular walking routine and was able to lose her excess pounds without ever bullying herself.

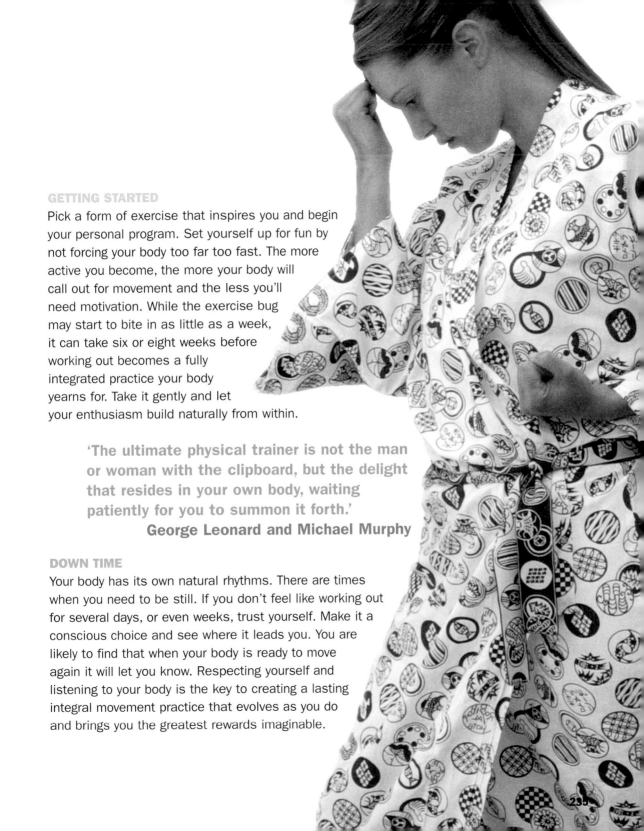

GETTING STARTED

Pick a form of exercise that inspires you and begin
your personal program. Set yourself up for fun by
not forcing your body too far too fast. The more
active you become, the more your body will
call out for movement and the less you'll
need motivation. While the exercise bug
may start to bite in as little as a week,
it can take six or eight weeks before
working out becomes a fully
integrated practice your body
yearns for. Take it gently and let
your enthusiasm build naturally from within.

'The ultimate physical trainer is not the man
or woman with the clipboard, but the delight
that resides in your own body, waiting
patiently for you to summon it forth.'
George Leonard and Michael Murphy

DOWN TIME

Your body has its own natural rhythms. There are times
when you need to be still. If you don't feel like working out
for several days, or even weeks, trust yourself. Make it a
conscious choice and see where it leads you. You are
likely to find that when your body is ready to move
again it will let you know. Respecting yourself and
listening to your body is the key to creating a lasting
integral movement practice that evolves as you do
and brings you the greatest rewards imaginable.

CALL TO ACTION

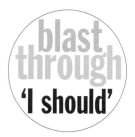

Make a Plan: Choose at least one activity to explore as an integral practice. Commit to doing it three times this week – ideally for 30 minutes each time. (If you are very unfit, start with a 10-minute practice and then work your way up.)

Dream It: Before you go to bed, visualize yourself enjoying whatever activity you have chosen for the following day. Rehearsing your intention helps to clear resistance and build enthusiasm.

Get an Invocation: Use the Movement Mantra exercise to create your own inspiring invocation. Write it out and put it somewhere you will see it several times a day. Repeat it as you exercise to keep you focused on your goal.

Go Shopping: Make sure you have the equipment you need for your exercise practice, such as a good pair of trainers, swimming goggles, a personal stereo with music, or an exercise DVD.

Record It: Keep an account of the pay offs you experience from workouts in your Journal. For instance: 'I had so much energy after my walk today… My skin looks great… I feel happier…' Refer back to your Journal entries to keep incentive strong.

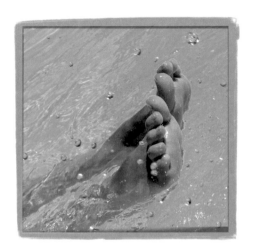

'Inner beauty is priceless. Outer
beauty doesn't have to be.'
Paula Begoun

16 GET HIGH

overdose and thrive

Being beautiful means getting high on life. There is bliss in the most unexpected places. You can reach levels of vitality, joy, clarity and freedom that you may only have dreamed of. All you need is savvy, a little help here and there and the determination to do it *your* way.

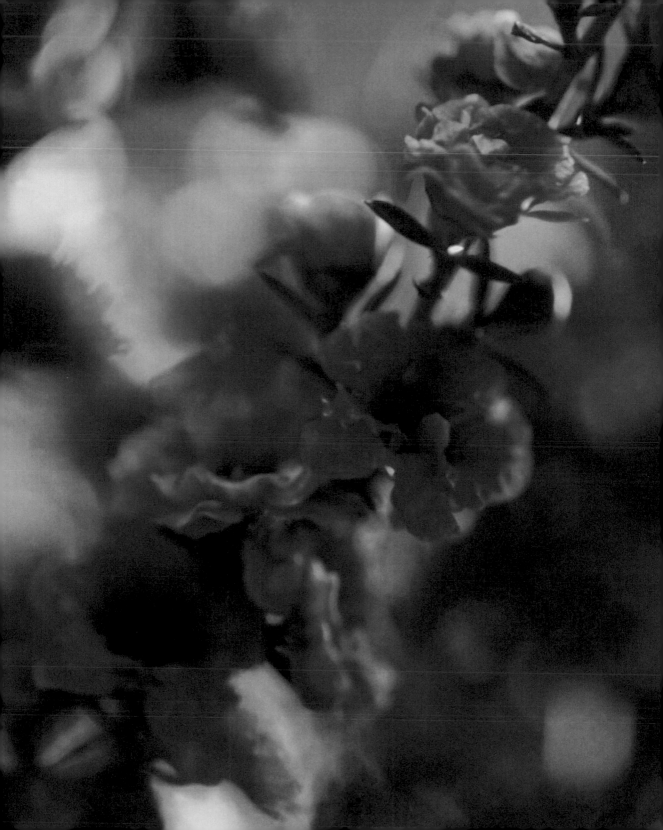

In our world of prescription drug pushers and nonsense advertising, getting high on life – the most exciting high in the universe, by the way – can be a challenge. Dig for information. Find what works for *you*. Be willing to change when life calls for it. Discriminating between truth and nonsense in the media, paying attention to your body's response to what you eat and how you live and think are all part of going for exhilaration. You can create your own reality; indeed, life exhilaration depends on it.

You do not need to follow everything you have read in this book – there would be no time to live any life at all if you did! In this chapter as in all others, make use of the things that appeal to you and leave the rest – you may find them useful at another time or you may never need them at all. It's your call.

You Are an Open System

Energetically your *body cum psyche* forms what is known as an *open system*. It continually exchanges information, order, biochemistry and energy with its environment – through the foods you eat, digest and assimilate, as well as the water you drink, the air you breathe, the feelings you feel and thoughts you think, even the company you keep.

Electromagnetic and subtle energies you are exposed to also take part in the exchange. As such we are constantly processing mechanical, biochemical and energetic *information* which comes to us and flows from us. To thrive we need a constant supply of the *right kind* of information from the outside world. This keeps our lives on track and helps us function optimally. We also need to *dissipate disorder* – to get rid of the waste and chaos that builds up in our bodies and psyches – radiation from computers and mobile phones, sounds, people's moods, energy fields themselves. Here's the equation: take in information with a high level of order and eliminate the rubbish efficiently, then your whole life works better. But when the processes of energy exchange fall down on either count, we're in trouble.

> 'The scientific theory I like best is that the rings of Saturn are composed entirely of lost airline luggage.'
>
> **Mark Russell**

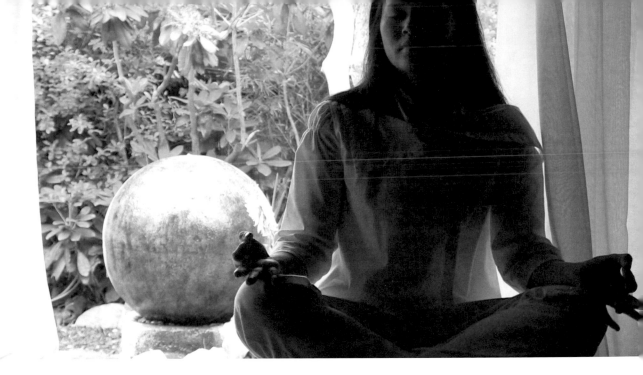

GO FOR IT

Clean water, fresh air, good food and plenty of laughter establish radiant well-being and help you heal when things get out of sync. Laughter? Right. It's just about the best medicine in the world. Laughter gets your breathing going. It makes hormones flow. Laughter even improves your immune system. Find humour in your day-to-day existence, especially when all around you things seem to be falling apart, and you will have discovered a major secret of the universe. Laughter brings a sense of detachment. It protects us from getting lost in minutiae. It helps us sail through onslaughts of fear, guilt, resentment, anger and embarrassment, which plague us all from time to time.

DVD THERAPY

We love the movies. Leslie, especially, is a complete film fanatic. Great movies to make you laugh are hard to come by. Here are a few of our favourites:

- Dirty Rotten Scoundrels ● Bowfinger ● Mickey Blue Eyes
- Don Juan De Marco ● Bringing Up Baby ● Nothing to Lose
- A Fish Called Wanda ● Bullets Over Broadway ● I Love You To Death
- Roxanne ● The Producers ● To Be or Not to Be

Hydroelectric Turn On

The oldest system of natural healing in the world uses hot and cold baths and showers to increase vitality, balance hormones, beautify skin, tone muscles, clear the mind, vitalize nerves and improve circulation. It quickly turns on your aliveness, all the while dissolving, transporting and clearing rubbish from body and psyche, thereby further heightening your vitality.

Thanks to water's chemical and bioelectrical properties, and to our body's physiological and energetic responses to them, water therapy is a great way to deep-cleanse, energize and restore youthful functioning to a tired or ageing body. The technique of using alternating applications of hot and cold water is called 'Contrast Hydros'. After a workout, athletes use hydroelectrics in the form of contrast baths and showers to strengthen the body, prevent muscular damage and eliminate aches. If you have not yet experienced the turn on it offers, you have a real treat ahead.

THE PROTOCOLS

Using *hydroelectrics* is easy provided you are generally healthy and not suffering from a heart condition.

Apply hot water to your whole body for three or four minutes in the form of a hot bath or shower. Follow with 30 to 60 seconds of cold water. Repeat the procedure three times. The application of cold water needs to be just long enough to make blood vessels constrict. This can take place in as little as 20 seconds.

Cold water triggers the sympathetic nervous system to energize, while hot water intensifies parasympathetic activity for relaxation. The combination of the two makes you feel great. But start slowly, increasing the length of your exposure to hot and cold water gradually. If you have a separate bath and shower you can use the bath for one temperature application, the shower for the other, moving back and forth. During the summer, make your bath cold and your showers hot. During the winter reverse this.

Out of the silence came the song
out of the stillness came the dance
out of the darkness came colour.

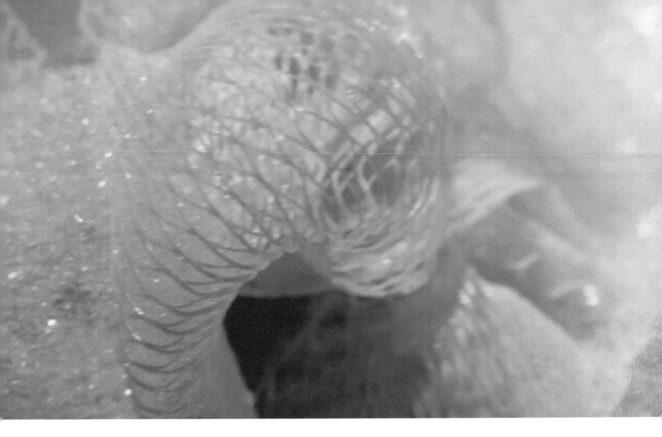

TRY SHEER INTENSITY

Like any natural treatment, contrast hydros need to be followed carefully and wisely to get all the benefits you can and to ensure that no harm is done. You will probably find, as Leslie did at first, that a plunge into cold water or a cold shower is a shock to the body. Soon, however, this turns into an experience of total pleasure.

- Don't use contrast hydros if you have any kind of heart condition, nervous disorder, high blood pressure, if you are an insulin-dependent diabetic or suffer from hardening of the arteries. Always check with your doctor before beginning any natural treatment to make sure that it is appropriate for you.

- Make sure your body is warm before beginning. The room should be well heated. Don't let your body become chilled during the treatment. If you feel yourself becoming too cold, immediately stop and get into a hot bath or shower until you warm up fully.

- Always begin with a hot application and end with cold. Start slowly with 2-3 minutes of hot application followed by 20 seconds of cold. As your body gets used to contrast hydros, increase the time of the cold applications up to 1 minute (even up to 2-3 minutes if you are extremely fit or an athlete).

- When you finish, dry your body well and dress warmly.

Internal Hydroelectrics

Another way to get high on energy is to drink plenty of pure water. When you give your body enough clean water it becomes energized. Circulation works better as does lymphatic drainage. You become less bothered by cellulite. Ironically, drinking plenty of clean water helps eliminate water retention in the tissues. When your body is short of water – and few of us drink enough – it holds wastes and fluids in the tissues, undermining energy, making your skin and muscles puffy and spoiling the natural contours of your face and body.

HOW MUCH DO YOU NEED

Drink enough water that your urine is pale in colour. For most women that's the equivalent of about 8-10 large glasses a day. Part of your daily quota can come from herb teas or natural juices made from fresh fruits and vegetables. (Coffee doesn't count. It is dehydrating.) However you choose to take it, clean water is essential for continually detoxifying the body, keeping the intestinal tract clean and bringing you high levels of energy and long-term stamina.

KEEP IT CLEAN

Clear, clean water can be hard to find. Tap water is seldom totally safe. Urban water is an unnatural, highly processed substance. It contains many chemical additives and contaminants. This makes spring water the best choice, provided you pick a water whose origins are known and which has been tested and certified clean. This is where the French waters come in. The control that is exerted over the quality of spring water in France is higher than any other place in the world. One of the best spring waters is Volvic, an exceptionally pure, still, variety from the Auvergne mountains in Central France.

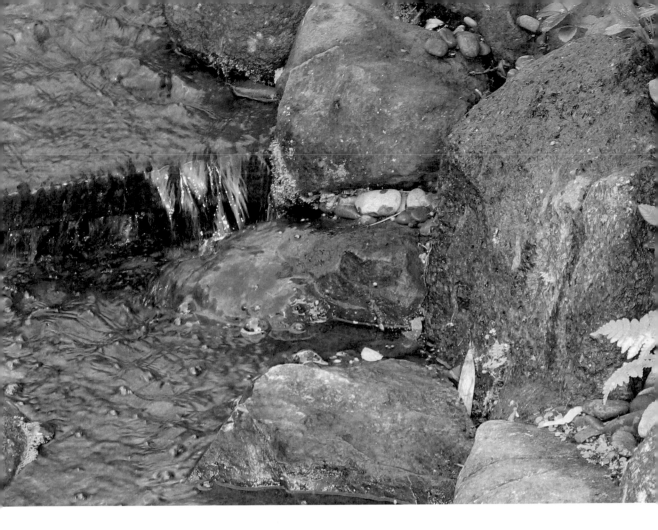

FILTER IT CLEAN

Home water filters vary in effectiveness. Solid carbon filters will not remove fluoride, but are fine for taking out chlorine, parasites, chemicals, and some heavy metals. Reverse osmosis filters don't remove chlorine unless you also use a carbon filter. But they will take out fluorides, parasites, bacteria, chemicals, as well as heavy metals and some of the basic minerals (most of which you would be better off leaving in). Distillation removes practically everything except possibly a few toxic chemicals. But heavy-duty water purification systems can be expensive. A general rule, if your water supply is not too bad, is to use a simple portable water purification jug for the water that will be heated to cook foods, while drinking and making teas from (if you can afford it) a good French mineral water.

Let There Be Light

What about the food you eat? Here too you want to feed on life. More specifically for radiance and vitality you want to feed on *light*. Good nutrition is not only biochemical in nature. The state and quality of living energy in the foods you eat greatly determines the health of your capillaries and cells, the shine on your hair and the radiance of your skin. This is not surprising since your body is literally made out of light. Believe it or not, it's the same light that flared forth 13.7 billion years ago when the universe was born.

QUANTUM HEALTH AND BEAUTY

Fresh, live plants – fruits and vegetables, seeds and herbs – carry a special form of light energy directly derived from the sun during photosynthesis. Provided they are grown on healthy organic soils in unpolluted air and clean water, they carry the highest levels of light energy and energetic order. They in turn convey the highest levels of order to our bodies when we eat them. Lasting, radiant health and beauty demands a high level of such order.

An apple, a leaf of lettuce, a grape, a sprout of rice, holds a high level of living. When we eat them, this life energy becomes available to our bodies, feeding our own vitality. A plant's ability to convey to those who eat it the highest levels of light-enhancing power depends on two things: clean air from the atmosphere and minerals and trace elements from the soil. From air, the plant extracts nitrogen and carbon dioxide, allowing it to capture light in the form of photons for growth and storage. From the soil they extract minerals to support their structure and light-gathering processes. When the soils on which a food is grown are depleted of minerals, trace elements and contaminated with pesticides and herbicides, the plant's growth and nature become distorted, increasing free radical generation and damage. This damage is transferred to us when we eat them. Plants need to be either completely unprocessed or at least minimally processed to help us when we eat them to get high on life. Processing and overcooking destroys the lion's share of the biochemical and energetic information we need in order to live in a state of optimal health.

'If anything is sacred, the human body is sacred.'
Walt Whitman

Be Still

Getting high on life is not simply a question of revving up, it is just as much about revving down. Simply being still and finding a place of real joy can be one of the greatest highs that life has to offer.

The word 'God' is distasteful to some. Little wonder, since we've been raised with the notion we're supposed to believe in an invisible being who sits in Heaven and looks a bit like Santa Claus, who rewards us if we're good and punishes us when we're bad. Drop any idea of God that does not ring true for you. Develop your own sense of the divine, the wonderment of life, the unexplainable, whatever inspires you. Then with a little practice, you can learn to draw on this energy to manifest whatever you choose, from the deepest levels of your being. Made popular in recent years by a few Cistercian friars and others including writers and thinkers such as William Meninger, Basil Pennington and Thomas Keating, Centring Prayer bears little resemblance to what is generally thought of as prayer. It makes no requests of God or anyone else and it carries no agendas. Instead, it uses a silently repeated sacred word expressing your intention to open yourself to the divine – beyond all thought, emotion and image.

PURE AWARENESS

Centring Prayer directs your attention from the outside world towards pure awareness within. In many ways this is akin to a Zen *koan* which, by silencing the mind, opens consciousness to a deeper awareness of reality. It can initiate big changes in your life. From a kind of spiritual detox where false ideas and old blockages clear, it can bring perfect realizations about life, the universe and everything. It is neither self-hypnosis, nor meditation, nor a form of relaxation. Its effects go beyond all three.

If you are Christian you might like to explore a particularly Christian approach which you will find instructions for in Father Thomas Keating's book *Open Mind, Open Heart*. But you can be Christian, Buddhist, Muslim, Agnostic – even an atheist – and still tap into its transformative power. It is so simple. You enter interior silence and allow it to do whatever it will. All you need is a sacred word, a comfortable seat and twenty minutes.

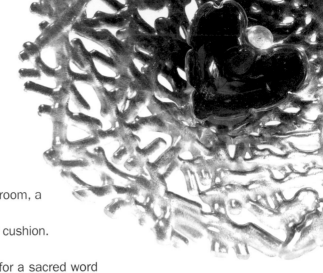

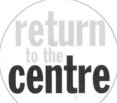

return to the centre

● Find a quiet place – a room, a park, a church, a car.
● Sit upright on a chair or cushion. Relax.
● Close your eyes and ask for a sacred word that represents your intention to merge with whatever you consider the highest reality – God, Nature, Great Spirit, the Universe, the deepest levels of your own soul. Your word could be 'One' or 'Beloved' or 'Love.' Whatever you choose it should feel good to you and carry a sense of wonder. (You'll use the same word each time.)

● Begin *very gently* to repeat your sacred word. You are likely to discover that in time, the word begins to repeat itself of its own accord. The word seems to dissolve away as you pass over the threshold of stillness. That's fine.

● When distracting thoughts, feelings or noises arise, gently bring your awareness back to repeating your sacred word.

● After 20 minutes end your practice. An alarm clock with a pleasant-sounding chime can be useful. Otherwise, gently check your watch to see when 20 minutes is up.

● Give yourself a minute or two to come back.

● Open your eyes.

TRUE TRANSFORMATIONS

The changes which take place when you commit yourself to using this type of practice are *discontinuous* in nature. They appear to happen out of nowhere. In reality a lot of inner changes have been happening before major shifts in your day-to-day life become evident. The growing sense of greater freedom, joy and meaning that develop in time are *not simple changes*. They are true *transformations* – passages out of a *limited* way of being into a more *expanded* one.

NOW – NOT THEN OR WHEN

Developing your ability to live 'in the *now*' is important to ending chronic discontent with life and opening to joy. Our thoughts constantly pull us out of the now, into the future or the past. The past is often burdened with regret about what we did or didn't do. The future is frequently laden with anxiety about what may or may not happen. *Now* simply *is*. As we begin to develop a sense of who we are beyond the thinking mind – the aim of Return to the Centre – we experience more freedom. Spiritual teacher Eckhart Tolle speaks and writes wonderfully about living in the now. Any practice that brings you into the present moment – from sensuous delight in a fragrance, to meditation, prayer or rock climbing – brings a sense of freedom and awakens an experience of joy in living right here, right now.

'Nothing in all creation is so like God as stillness.'
Meister Eckhart

Electronic Transformation

Want more quantum leaps, faster? Electronically created binaural technology has something significant to offer. Leslie has used it for several years.

ENLIGHTENING SOUNDS

Binaural technology comes in the form of CDs or tapes which you listen to when you relax, meditate or pray. Binaurals use advanced neuro-audio techniques which enable the listener to enter a desirable state by shifting brainwave frequencies out of *beta* – our usual state of awareness – into the deeper *alpha, theta and delta*, each of which brings its own benefits. The best of these CDs uses various frequencies in specific progressive ways. They are designed to link up disparate parts of the brain, thereby enhancing neurological functions. Using binaural technology daily can lead to better sleep, a greater capacity to handle stress, and improved health. It can also bring about emotional and spiritual development. Some of the best programmes are designed in a step-by-step way. You use one set of CDs or tapes for, say, three or four months, then move on to the next, so that neurological changes take place in an ordered and progressive way. Simpler programmes are also available (see Resources).

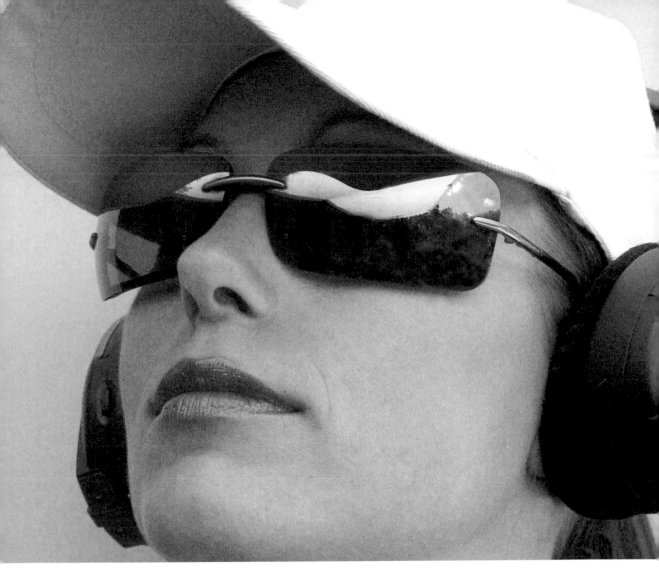

POWERS TO TRANSFORM

Laughter, moving the body, listening to the whispers of your soul and honouring your dreams – all these things breed high levels of power for transformation. Illness and degeneration happen when we become prey to energy blockages, imbalances and leakage, all of which siphon off natural vitality, distort metabolic functions and undermine belief in ourselves and our life. Finding stillness, making use of hydro-electric stimulation and bringing more light energy into the food you eat are all ways that can help recreate an ordered, harmonious flow of life energy, which in turn contribute greatly to the process of becoming who you really are.

CALL **TO** ACTION

Get Hysterical: Feed on fun by watching a film that makes you laugh uncontrollably.

Shower Boost: Start the day on a high, or revive yourself for a night out with a contrast hydros shower.

Water High: Keep a plentiful supply of clean, pure water on hand. Buy a filter, if necessary, or stock up on bottled water. Keep your energy levels high by staying well hydrated throughout the day.

Eat Light: Shop for the finest, simplest foods, filled with light and beauty that will feed you in the best possible ways.

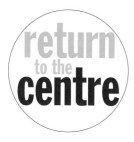

Your Secret Word: Take five minutes this week to sit down, light a candle, close your eyes and become still. Ask for a word that can help you experience your connection with the divine. See what comes. When you find the word that is right for you, you'll know.

Brain Wave Massage: Consider investing in one of the binaural technology CDs and use it regularly to access expanded awareness.

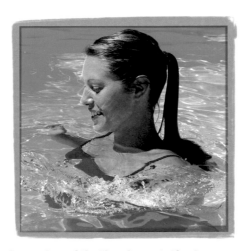

'It is only with the heart that one can
see rightly; what is essential is
invisible to the eye.'
Antoine de Saint-Exupery

17 LIFE MAKEOVER

past...present...future

Our lives are made up of stories – some we witness, some we choose to live out, others play themselves out without our choosing. The lens through which we view these stories determines our quality of life. Look at an experience – say a physical handicap – through one lens and you cast yourself in the role of the victim. Look at the same circumstance through another and you emerge as the hero.

> 'My life has been filled with terrible misfortune; most of which never happened.'
>
> **Montaigne**

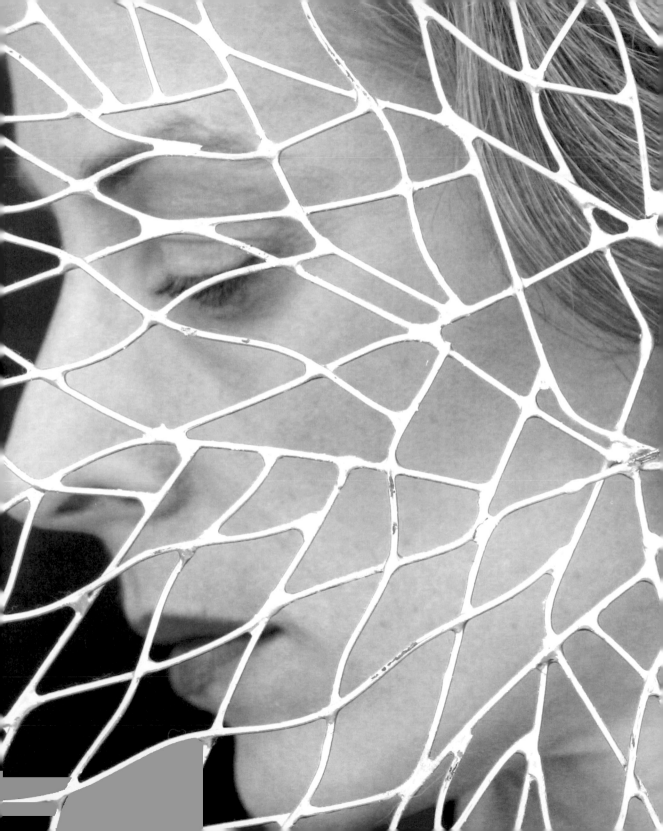

How you interpret your life's events can ensnare you or set you free. Deciding to change perspective can mean the difference between a life of disappointment and bitterness and one filled with joy and the deepest fulfilment possible. The choice lies with you.

A Fall to Grace – Leslie's Story

While boarding British Airways flight 949 from Munich to London, I had an accident which ripped my life asunder. I walked down a ramp running with water, slipped and fell onto my left knee, and split my leg open. Blood gushed everywhere. The other passengers were held at the gate while the cabin crew and I tried to stem the flow of blood.

In the midst of any disaster, surreal things happen. This was no exception. No sooner had we stopped the profuse flow of blood, than bizarre German paramedics arrived dressed in *combat gear*. One came up to me, grabbed my knee, and split the wound open again. 'You go to hospital immediately,' he barked. I told him that I was going home to London. I asked him to leave. He said, 'I will need your credit card then.' 'My credit card?' I said: 'No way am I giving you my credit card.' 'Then I call the Police,' he replied. At that point the pilot arrived. He announced, 'Go away, British Airways takes full responsibility.' Happily, they marched off.

Back in London, I was met by a wheelchair and taken home. I stayed in bed for a week since I couldn't walk. The wound itself healed, leaving only a small scar at the front of my knee. The knee was still swollen and painful, but I figured that would go away before long. Boy, was I ever wrong. Everything fell apart. The injury was the worst I've ever had, and three years later my body is still in the process of healing.

I did not know that when injury is bad enough, an accident can not only cause physical damage, it can undermine your immune system and diminish the way you view your life. In the first year that followed the fall, I came down with both pneumonia and measles.

The accident precipitated a cascade of physical injuries. Many resulted from the gross imbalance in the way I was forced to carry my body because of pain in my left leg. I couldn't walk for 18 months, I couldn't exercise and I gained 20 kilos in weight. Plunged into despondency when none of the treatments brought much relief, I was made powerless by my inability to help myself.

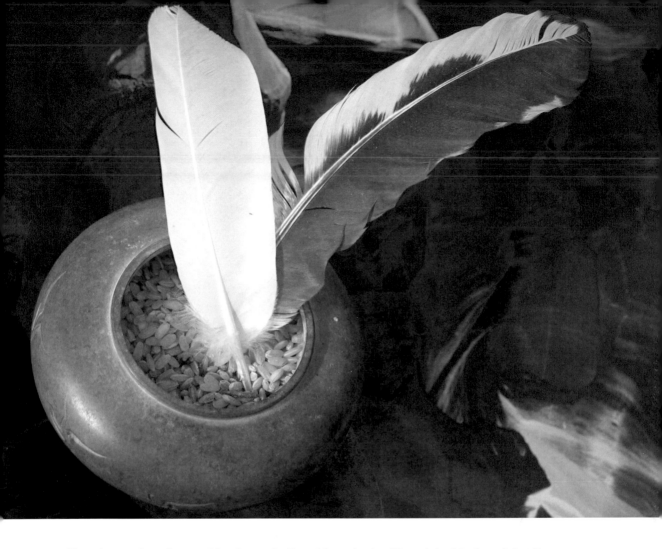

First, I questioned everything I ever believed in or had written. I doubted my integrity, my knowledge, my intelligence. Then I was plagued with thoughts like, 'Will I ever recover?' The accident forced me to look deeper into my own soul, to re-order my values and to get clear about what I wanted from the deepest levels of my being in relation to my work and my life. It forced me to do in-depth research in biochemistry, energetic medicine and advanced methods of natural healing. All the suffering resulting from it – and it is by no means over – has also awakened my senses and heightened my appreciation of beauty – like the smell of jasmine, the sound of water over rocks, a sunrise. It's showed me that, no matter what condition we are in, the richness of our lives – even lying flat on your back in bed where you can see nothing but a branch of a tree through a window – is so intense and wondrous we can't begin to express its beauty. For all this – including the pain, fear, despondency and confusion – I have, at last, become infinitely grateful.

'Pain is inevitable. Suffering is optional.'
Kathleen C. Theisen

Susannah's Story

When I began to work on this book I had just gone through a devastating break-up. The man I lived with, whom I believed was my life-long partner, left me, unable to explain why. Two weeks later I discovered he'd become involved with another woman. I dived headlong into the role of victim, lamenting the betrayal and mourning the loss of a relationship I had treasured. Friends and family supported and reinforced my position as the 'wronged woman'. I nursed my broken heart. But somehow victim-hood didn't sit well with me. It brought me no relief. I went through long months of grieving, forgiving (or trying to) and soul searching. Finally, I began to look at the separation through a new lens. I came to see that during the time I lived with my ex-partner I had sacrificed my creativity and self-expression to tend to his needs. My devotion to him, rather than allowing me to evolve, had kept me from moving forward. I saw that his choice to leave, guided by his new partner's allure, was part of a larger plan being orchestrated for my highest good and no doubt theirs too.

'Reality is always kinder than the stories we tell about it.'
Byron Katie

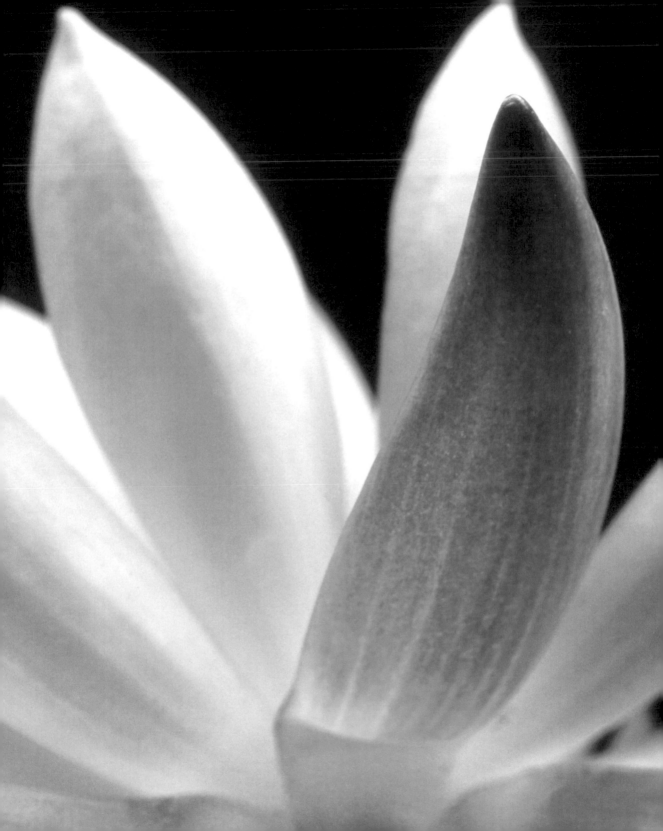

re-write your past

In her book, *Women Who Run With the Wolves*, Jungian analyst and storyteller Clarissa Pinkola Estés, describes an exercise she uses with clients called 'Descansos.' A Spanish word that means 'resting places', descansos also refers to the little crosses you see beside treacherous roads that mark the site of a fatal accident. Estés has her clients draw a timeline of their lives and mark it with descansos to represent the moments where 'deaths' have occurred. These deaths might be an actual death or the death of a dream. She then recommends clients mourn those incidents and lay them to rest.

We use a process similar to Estés as a first step in identifying moments in your life where 'deaths' have occurred. We then explore ways to transmute these experiences so that you can re-tell your life story for greater peace, joy and fulfilment.

Here's how:

Step One: Take a large sheet of paper and draw a horizontal line through the centre. Divide it up into ten-year sections: 0-10 years old, 11-20, 21-30 and so on. Then mark at the appropriate point in time any incident that occurred in your life that felt like a death. It might have been a divorce, the loss of a job, the death of a loved one, a betrayal, the end of a dream, an injury or illness, a miscarriage, an abortion, leaving a country you loved, turning down a proposal. Draw a cross and label each event.

Step Two: Now look at your crosses and feel your way into each of them. Find the sticking places – those events that still carry a strong emotional charge or weigh you down. Set the intention to clear residual trauma surrounding these events. One way to do this is with ritual. You might gather flower petals or leaves to represent your feelings about an event and release them into a flowing stream. Or you might write about your unresolved feelings in connection with what happened and then burn the pages. You could even write a letter of forgiveness to someone you feel betrayed by. Then choose to send it to them, or not – whichever is most appropriate and freeing.

Step Three: Next, gently explore the events on your time line as potential blessings. What gift, if any, have they brought you? In what way have they changed your life for the better? Record your discoveries in your Journal.

Each 'death' is in some way also a rebirth. It forces you to let go of things you may think you need, but which impede your expansion and the full expression of your authenticity. In the midst of anguish and grief it can be hard to remember this. In retrospect it becomes easier to understand that every hardship you face serves your unfolding. There is a tendency in all of us to define ourselves by the 'bad' things that happen. Doing this restricts you in every way. It's important to process any trauma and let it go so that you can define yourself in a new way.

After doing the above exercise, you're likely to discover, next time you speak about your past, that the story you tell is a very different one. The 'dreadful' childhood you have lamented for years may become a source of humour to you. Or you may discover a soft spot for a friend who betrayed you. The possible ways to retell your life story are infinite – the perspective you choose is up to you.

'In a very real sense we are the authors of our own lives.'
Mandy Aftel

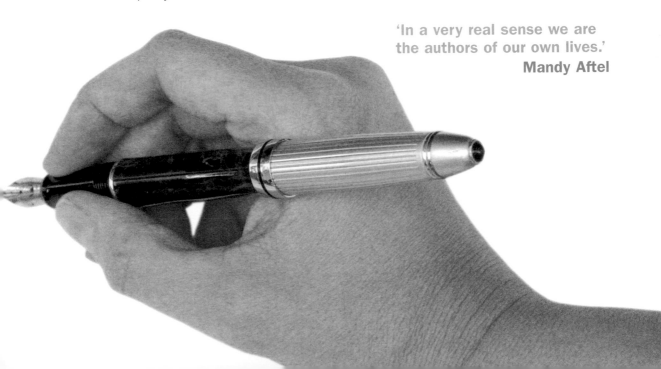

Live the Present

As you make peace with your past, you free yourself to live more in the present – even to celebrate it. Several of the integral practices in this book, such as Centring Prayer reinforce your ability to live in the *now*. So does becoming more fully *embodied* through conscious exercise and opening to greater levels of bliss. This is what the integrated practices in this book have been all about. The more you live in the moment, the more you are able to move beyond feelings of separation – from yourself and from others – and to experience your connection with all life.

Then, it becomes easier to sense for yourself what the great philosophers and mystics have always taught – that life is *for*, not *against*, you.

CRUISING CRISIS

It's easy to lose perspective in the midst of upheaval. Life can be tough: you get fired. Your best friend dies. You're diagnosed with cancer. You get pushed to your limits – and often beyond. Authentic living does not make you immune to crisis. Indeed, choosing the authentic path can even precipitate a crisis that has been brewing beneath the surface. As you refuse to adapt to systems that don't serve you, life re-shuffles things to enable you to come into your own. The process can be downright painful. Rebirth, like birth, is messy. But, when you begin to look at everything in your path as an opportunity to unfold into a fuller, richer expression of who you are, something amazing happens. Instead of resisting change, you begin to embrace it. Instead of lamenting, 'Why is this happening to *me*?' you ask the same question in quiet anticipation of something wonderful. You enter the eye of the storm, like a caterpillar going into the safety of its cocoon, and emerge renewed and transformed by every challenge you face.

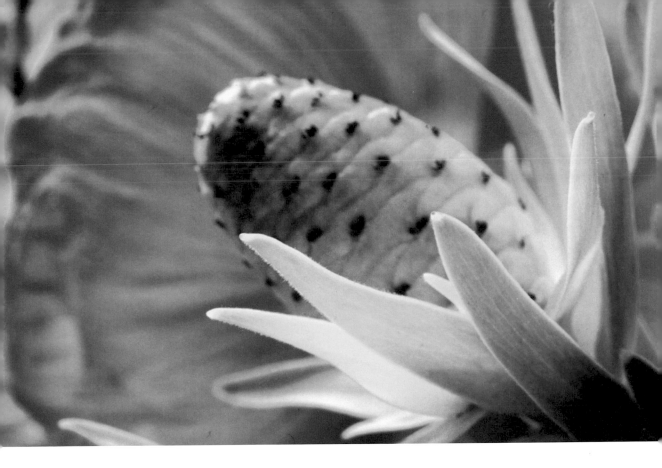

LESSONS FROM THE CATERPILLAR

Nature is a master of transformation. The humble caterpillar prepares to turn itself into a butterfly by building a cocoon. This sacred structure allows metamorphosis of the deepest order to occur safely. It's sacred because, whether it be hard and crisp or soft and flexible, a cocoon simply 'holds the space' while the powers of transformation encoded within every organism work their magic. They dissolve the caterpillar into a soft jelly. Then, knowing exactly what needs to happen from moment to moment, they reshape this jelly into the butterfly. Finally the newly born butterfly destroys the cocoon, which has served its purpose for protection in the midst of change, to emerge in all its glory.

Sacred space is a terrific ally as you navigate through crisis. Spin your own cocoon in non-ordinary reality. Enter its environment of wholeness and safety. Connect with your core, get healing and gather insights about yourself and your life. Call on the power of nature and emerge from your cocoon reborn.

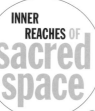

INNER REACHES OF sacred space

- Sit comfortably, or lie down, and close your eyes.
- Enter your Inner Reaches of Sacred Space.
- Activate your senses until you feel fully present in your special place.
- Call to the elements of nature for support – trees and grass, water and air, rocks, fire and earth.
- Call upon spirit helpers – animals, people, teachers, helpers, guides – whom you have met in your special place before, or who may show up for the first time now.
- Ask these spirits to weave a cocoon of safety and support around you to bring ease and grace to the challenge you face.
- Notice what happens when you do this. How does your body feel?
- Enjoy the blessings, love and support of these spirits by simply being in their presence for a few minutes.
- If you want guidance, ask for it now.
- Thank each spirit helper for its gifts and love.
- In your own time, gently bring your consciousness back to ordinary reality and open your eyes.

Record your experience and insights in your Journal as words, drawings or in any other way you choose. Even if the information you get doesn't seem to make sense, play with it and allow it to evolve in your consciousness. The wisdom of spirit is not always obvious to the rational mind, but the protection of your cocoon will continue to support you in the real world if you keep your mind and heart open.

'The world of reality has limits. The world of imagination is boundless.'

Jean-Jacques Rousseau

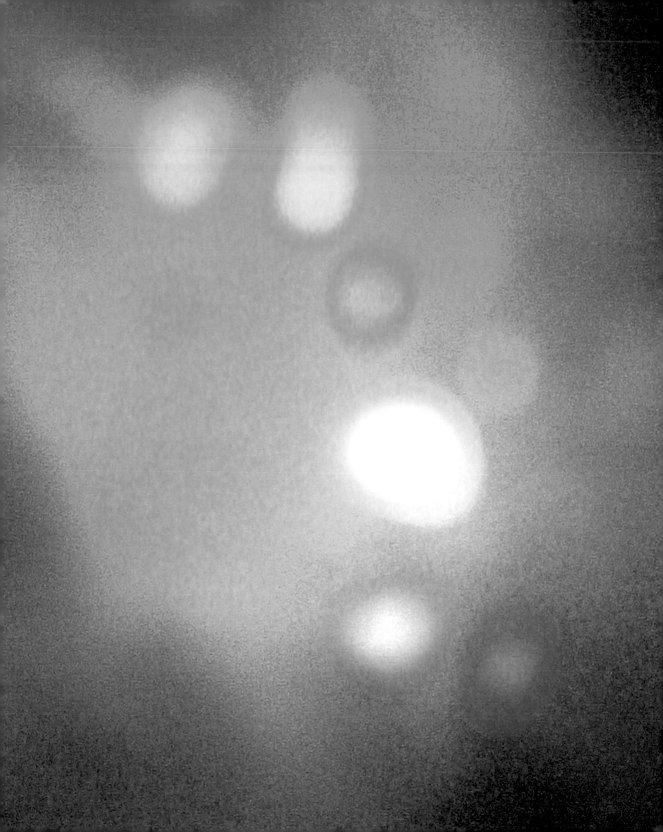

Take It to Bed

Just as cocooning in non-ordinary reality can support us through difficult times, so returning to the cocoon of your bed and getting plenty of sleep is essential to dealing with crisis. During sleep, your body repairs itself while your mind processes and orders your experience. Getting plenty of rest can give you the inner reserves of strength and resilience you need to deal with any challenge. More importantly, it is during sleep that profound transformation and shifts in consciousness occur. When you deprive yourself of sleep, you stunt your personal and spiritual growth.

Studies show most adults do best with six to eight hours of sleep a night. (Teenagers may need 9 and young children up to 12 hours.) Adequate sleep also prevents premature ageing, bringing us the mental and physical vitality we need to deal with crisis.

SLEEP YOURSELF YOUNGER

A study published in *The Lancet* in October 1999, concluded that sleep deprivation may hasten the onset of age-related illnesses, including diabetes, hypertension and memory loss. Researchers studied 11 healthy young men for 16 nights. The first three nights the men were allowed to sleep eight hours. The next six nights they slept just four hours and the final seven nights they spent twelve hours in bed. After several nights of sleep deprivation, the men's ability to regulate glucose/insulin levels (one of the biomarkers for age) had decreased by 30 per cent.

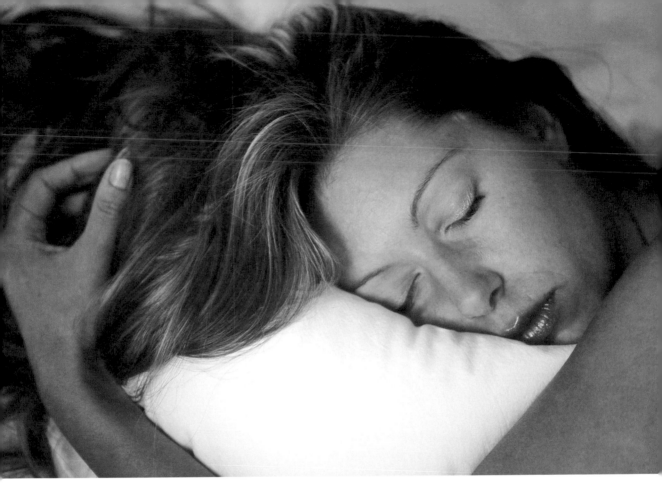

SLEEP HELPERS

Make use of the following tips to banish insomnia, promote blissful sleep and awaken refreshed with a whole new outlook on life:

● **Blackout:** Make your bedroom as dark as possible. Exposure to light at night inhibits the secretion of melatonin – a pineal-gland hormone – needed to regulate circadian rhythms, promote healthy cell growth and induce restful sleep.

● **Sleepy Snack:** Avoid grains and sugars right before going to bed. They can cause a 'sugar-high-sugar-low' reaction that can wake you up several hours later. If you want a snack, opt for one high in the calming amino acid L-tryptophan – a slice of turkey breast, a handful of almonds or a banana.

● **Herbal Tranquility:** Use relaxing herbs in the form of teas or tinctures to soothe body and mind. We especially like a product called SedaPlus by Thorne, as well as Celestial Seasoning's Sleepy Time Tea.

● **Damp Socks:** After a warm, relaxing bath take a pair of light cotton socks and dip them in cold water, wring them out as much as you can. Put them on your feet and cover them with a pair of dry socks, preferably woollen ones. This great hydrotherapy trick pulls your energy downwards, helping you drift off to sleep.

● **Slumber Waves:** When you're tired, but your mind is racing, call on binaural technology to shift brainwaves and drop you into sleep (see Resources).

● **Cut Interference:** If you sleep badly in your bedroom, see what you can do to reduce electromagnetic stress. Clear TVs, computers, electric alarm clocks and electric blankets from your room. Second best, unplug them.

● **Restful Chi:** Arrange your bedroom furniture so that when lying in bed you can see the door. Ideally, according to feng shui law, the door should be diagonally opposite you. Avoid having a window, mirror or doorway behind your head.

● **Early To Bed:** The body, including the adrenals, does much of its recharging between the hours of 11pm and 1am. If you are still awake at this time, toxins tend to buid up in your liver, making you even more tired. Get to bed by 10pm whenever you can.

● **Nap Up:** If you don't manage to get your 8 hours of sleep, don't panic. A power nap of as little as 10-20 minutes in the late afternoon can help undo much of the damage of sleep deprivation.

'Sleep knits up the ravell'd sleeve of care.'
William Shakespeare

Niggling Dissatisfaction

It's not just the big challenges in life that undermine well-being. Feeling chronically discontented or low subtly erodes the quality of your day-to-day reality. Here, too, you have a say in the matter. There are simple things you can do to help brighten your outlook, shift perspective and tap into more joy.

PLUNGE INTO GRATITUDE

Resentment is a joy-killer. It casts a shadow over all you do, separates you from happiness and makes life miserable.

Next time you feel unhappy, stop and count your blessings. Really. Although it may be the last thing you feel like doing, tapping the power of gratitude can quickly dissolve resentment and anger, melt away a sense of 'poor me' and help realign you with life's blessings.

Write down, or speak aloud, five things you are grateful for, such as:

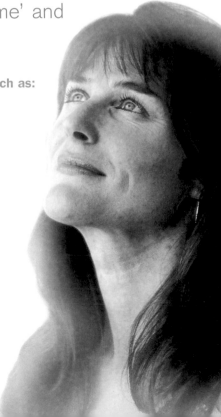

I am grateful for…
- The tree outside my window.
- The email I just received from my friend.
- Freshly squeezed orange juice.
- My accountant.
- Stevie Wonder's music.

If five things don't get your gratitude flowing, think of five more. Keep going until the sense of true thanksgiving kicks in. If you're going through a particularly tough time, begin and end each day by making a gratitude list in your Journal. It's powerful medicine for transformation.

Create Your Future

Throughout this book we've explored ways to get to know and express more of your authentic self. We've looked at ways to enhance natural beauty and expand bliss, to clear limiting beliefs, fill your body with more light, build more power into your muscles. You may even have begun to trust your ability to shift material reality through focused intention. Now let's have some fun putting it all together. Map out your authentic self in all its splendour and set intentions for the future you want to create.

'Just trust yourself, then you will know how to live.'

Goethe

MANIFESTATION BOARD GAME

We both have *Manifestation Boards* hanging in our bedrooms. We made them together one evening and regularly re-work them, adding new intentions and inspirational pictures or quotes. We highly recommend this exercise, done alone or with friends. It is a powerful way to focus your intentions and help turn your dreams and desires into realities.

You'll need:

- A large white board/piece of card
- Colourful paper
- Pens, crayons, pastels, etc.
- Scissors
- Bluetack and/or tape
- Pictures that inspire you.
- Brightly coloured ribbons, stickers, stars, glitter.

Establish sacred space with a simple ritual, such as lighting a candle and taking three deep breaths. Your intention is to delve deeply into your heart's desires and create symbols for their manifestation in your life.

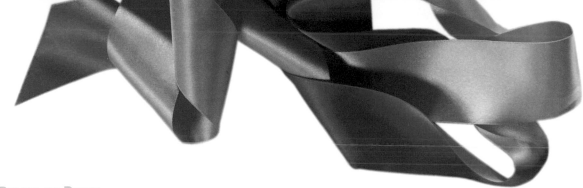

Dream on Paper

Write down your dreams, desires and goals on individual pieces of paper. Don't limit yourself or edit out a dream that feels impossible – get each one down. Consider areas such as your career, family, health, spiritual development, beauty, creativity, abundance, travel, education, relationships, community and play.

As you write your dreams and goals, put them in the present tense as if they already exist. In other words, not 'I want to buy a home in Tuscany' but 'I own a home in Tuscany'. Passion empowers manifestation, so the more passionate you are about the goals you set the better. In addition to goals, write down qualities you would like to embody, such as strength, compassion or boldness.

Conjure Images

Next, choose images that inspire and delight you. They can be related to your goals, but they needn't be. Cut them out of magazines, photocopy them from books, draw/paint them yourself or download them from the Internet.

Assemble your words and images on your white board. As you do, notice the relationship between the different elements. Be aware of your thoughts as you play with the pieces, arranging them in a way that inspires you. What do you notice? Are you excited by what you see emerging? Frustrated? Inhibited? Record whatever feelings come up in your Journal. If you are doing the exercise with friends, share your experiences.

Once you've arranged your board in a way that feels right, bluetack or tape your pieces in place. Find a spot for the board where you will see it every day. Keep interacting with it. Add or remove elements, alter an intention, shift a goal to a different spot, connect your pieces in a new way, infuse the board with more colour. Let it evolve as you do and enjoy the process.

'Twenty years from now you will be more disappointed by the things you didn't do than by the ones you did do. So throw off the bowlines. Sail away from the safe harbor. Catch the trade winds in your sails. Explore. Dream. Discover.'

Mark Twain

We Stand Beside You

We stand poised at the beginning of a new millennium. It's a time for healing and of new beginnings – a time of great horror in the world filled with the hungry and the dying, pollution and loss, but also of great promise. Something is in the air. Women everywhere sense it. A new world of possibilities is being born.

We believe that the more each of us gains access to our wisdom and our creativity, our vision and our compassion – the more we will be able to work together with respect for all to create a world of beauty, balance and joy. As women we need balance, vision, clarity of mind, strong bodies and determination to love our truth. We need practice at focusing our intention and accessing our freedom. Such gifts are never found in religious or political systems, in philosophies or psychological ideas. The very best of their teaching may inspire us to open up our thinking in a way that sparks our own creative ideas and urges us to delve deeper and dream vaster dreams for our future. But the real power out of which we can create the future lies not outside us, but within the individual soul of each and every woman.

Access your freedom and your authentic power.

Speak your truth.

Live your bliss.

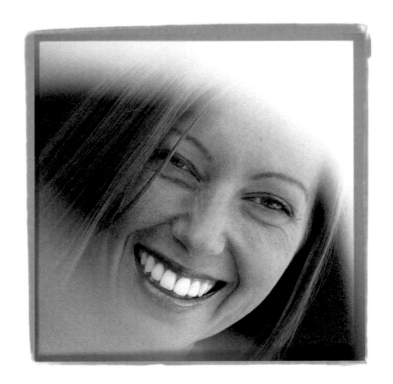

We stand
right beside you,
cheering.

Resources

Authentic Woman Website:
www.Authentic-Woman.com
The Authentic Woman process does not stop with this book. Be sure to visit the Authentic Woman website where you will find a wealth of inspiring information designed to help you on your journey towards becoming your authentic self. There you will find an Authentic Woman Workshop including practical exercises and audio files; techniques for finding your authentic voice; and much more.

Further reading:
There are some wonderful books that can inspire and guide you in your own authentic process. We have included a list of them on the Authentic Woman website

Leslie Kenton's Website:
www.lesliekenton.com Packed with helpful information, tools, techniques, inspiration and resources.

USEFUL TOOLS AND GADGETS

Binaural Audio Technology CDs
These CDs are useful for accessing deep meditative states. Designed to be listened to with stereo headphones, they send different signals to each ear, altering brain wave patterns. The noise you actually hear sounds like rain. The most sophisticated, designed to be listened to in a progressive series are created by HolosyncH Audio Technology: Available in the UK and Europe from:

Lifetools
12 Tilbury Close
Caversham
Reading
Berkshire RG4 5JF
Tel: +44 (0) 1189 483 444
Website: **www.lifetools.com**

From other countries contact:
Centerpointe Research Institute
4720 SW Washington Street
Suite #104
Beaverton
OR 97005
USA.
Telephone +1 (800) 945 2741.
Website: **www.centerpointe.com**
A simpler, less expensive version of the binaural technology, is available from Awakened Minds. Their Insight CD includes three 24-minute tracks for meditation/deep relaxation. Their Focus 2-CD set contains a 72-minute track that can be used while exercising, a 50-minute track to heighten attention while working and a 22-minute track to boost creativity.

Awakened Minds Inc
PO Box 16604
Tampa
FL 33687-6604
USA
Tel: +1 (813) 569 7770
www.awakenedminds.com

Essential Oils
For good quality essential oils contact:

Essentially Oils Ltd
8,9,10 Mount Farm
Junction Road
Churchill
Chipping Norton
Oxfordshire OX7 6NP
UK
Tel: +44 (0) 1608 659 544
Fax: +44 (0) 1608 659 522

The Fragrant Earth Company Ltd
PO Box 182
Taunton
Somerset TA1 1YR
Tel: +44 (0) 1823 335 734
Fax: +44 (0) 1823 322 566

Tisserand Aromatherapy
Newtown Road
Hove
Sussex BN3 7BA
UK
Tel: +44 (0) 1273 325 666

Facial Flex
This facial muscle exerciser can be ordered from **www.Folica.com**
Tel: +1 (888) 919 4247

Far Infrared Sauna
Infrared saunas are ideal for detoxing the body and for easing aches and pains.

In the UK:
MagMed Ltd.
3 Willetts Court
Pottergate
Norwich NR2 1DG
UK
Tel: +44 (0) 845 22 55 008
Fax: +44 (0) 870 43 20 406
Website: **www.physiotherm.co.uk**

In the Asia Pacific Region:
MagMed Ltd
100 Munro Road
RD5 Tauranga
New Zealand
Tel: +64 (7) 552 4877
Fax: +64 (7) 552 4850
E-mail: **infor@magmed.oco.nz**
Website: **www.4sauna.co.nz**

Mandolin

Our favourite mandolin grater for salad making is made in Germany by Börner. You can order the 'Swissmar Borner V-Slicer Plus' online from **www.Amazon.com.**

Power Plate

Check online for gyms and salons near you that offer Power Plate. For further information contact the importer:

UK, Ireland and Australia
Power Plate UK
Liberation Fitness Systems Ltd
UK
Tel: +44 (0) 207 272 0770
E-mail: **sales@power-plateuk.com**

North America
Power Plate North America Inc
3363 Commercial Avenue
Northbrook IL 60062
USA
Tel: +1 (847) 509 6000
Fax: +1 (847) 509 6004
E-mail: **info@powerplateusa.com**

New Zealand
Level 6
5-7 Kingdon Street
Newmarket
Aukland
New Zealand
Tel: +64 (9) 521 4745
Fax: +64 (9) 521 5746
E-mail: **info@power-plate.co.nz**

Weight Training

If you're keen to get started on a strength training program, we recommend Michael Colgan's book: *The New Power Program – Protocols for Maximum Strength.* Vancouver:

Apple Publishing Company, 2001. Also, Karen Andes' *A Woman's Book of Strength.* Perigee Books, 1995. The following videos are useful, although they're available only in VHS-NTSC format. Unless you have a multi-system player, you may not be able to view them:

In Shape With Rachel McLish: Includes two excellent workouts – one for the upper and one for the lower body that use just a pair of dumbbells. A solid beginner/intermediate-level workout.

Shaping Up With Weights for Dummies by Tracy York: Includes 12 basic free weights exercises as well as stretching.

Keys to Weight Training for Men and Women by Bill Pearl: Includes three training routines with free weights. Designed to help you learn correct form.

NUTRITIONAL SUPPLEMENTS, HERBS & HELPERS

Functional Medicine

If you want to use nutritional supplements on your path to greater health and authenticity you cannot do better than to work with a doctor or other health practitioner specifically trained in functional medicine. This is a cutting-edge science-based healthcare approach where the underlying causes of illness are assessed and treated. Check out the Institute of Functional Medicine on the Web. Thorne Research and Metagenics are two of the best nutritional supplement companies whose products are sold through practitioners. They are also available from the Nutri Centre in London.

The Nutri Centre

The best suppliers of nutritional supplements and information, unique in the world. Many of the products mentioned in this book are available from them, including land-based coral minerals from Okinawa. The NutriCentre also has one of the finest collections of books on holistic health and nutrition including spiritual and psychological books related to health. This small shop in the basement of The Hale Clinic is always at the cutting edge of what is happening in holistic health. Their products can be ordered easily online or by telephone. The NutriCentre carries more than 20,000 health and natural beauty care products including those which are available in health food stores as well as those sold only through practitioners. What you order is dispatched within 24 hours throughout the world. They have become Britain's largest supplier of complementary medicine textbooks to British colleges and universities. They print an interesting newsletter on holistic health with extracts printed online. The center is dedicated to service. No order is too small or too large. Almost all of what you need for natural health and beauty you will find here. We can't recommend them highly enough.

7 Park Crescent
London W1B 1PF
UK
Tel: +44 (0) 207 436 5122
E-mail:
customerservices@nutricentre.com
Website: **www.nutricentre.com**

Oliver's Wholefood Store

Another excellent place which offers a full range of supplements and natural remedies with an efficient nationwide mail order service is Oliver's Wholefood Store. Full organic grocer with off-licence, specialising in excellent quality organic food – vegetables, fish, meat etc. Oliver's organise regular health lectures. You can also get natural household cleaners here (and at other good health food emporiums).

5 Station Approach
Kew Gardens
Richmond
Surrey
TW9 3QB
Tel: +44 (0) 208 948 3990
Fax: +44 (0) 208 948 3991
E-mail: info@oliverswholefoods.co.uk

Thorne Research

We use Thorne nutritional products more than any other brand. They are excellent in terms of quality, formulation and performance. We especially recommend their multivitamin and mineral supplement, 'Extra Nutrients.'

UK:

Interlink House

Asfordby Business Park
Melton Mowbray
Leicestershire
LE14 3JL
Tel: +44 (0) 1664 810 011
Fax: +44 (0) 1664 810 012
Email: info@health-interlink.co.uk
Website: www.health-interlink.co.uk

Australia

Graeme H Wallace

Unit 1 13 Elizabeth Street
PO Box 230
Bullen
VIC 3105
Tel: +61 (3) 984 87890
Fax: +61 (3) 984 87839

New Zealand

FX Med

2 Dunlop Road
PO Box 19033
Onekawa Napier
Tel: +64 (6) 843 9370
Fax: +64 (6) 843 9260
Website: fxmed.co.nz

Metagenics

UK:
Nutri Limited
Tel: +44 (0) 166 374 6559
Fax: +44 (0) 166 375 0590

Metagenics UK
Tel: +44 (0) 149 833 243
Fax: +44 (0) 149 833 254
Email: info@metagenics.co.uk

Australia

Health World Limited

Tel: +61 (7) 3260 3300
Fax: +61 (7) 3260 3399
Website: www.metagenics.com.au

New Zealand:

J.M. Marketing Ltd

2/15 Parkway Drive
Mairingi Bay
Auckland
NZ
Tel: +64 (9) 478 2540
Fax: +64 (9) 478 2740
Website: www.metagenics.co.nz

Xynergy Health Products

They specialise in selling the finest green nutritional products – such as spirulina and cereal grasses – you can buy. They also sell the only fully natural multiple vitamin and mineral formula derived from plants, called Pure Synergy™ a mix of 62 organically grown superfoods working together synergistically to support life-energy in its purest form. Vita Synergy for women and Vita Synergy for men is the first truly 100% all natural vitamin, mineral and herbal supplement made entirely from food source nutrients. It is highly bio-available. Xynergy products are available in sophisticated health food stores or can be ordered by post direct from them.

Xynergy Health Products

Elsted
Midhurst
West Sussex GU29 0JT
UK
Tel: +44 (0) 1730 813 642
Fax: +44 (0) 1730 815 109
email: naturally@xynergy.co.uk
Website: www.xynergy.co.uk

Solgar Vitamin & Herb

An American company founded in 1947 which produces good quality nutritional supplements and standardised single herbs and formulas under strict pharmaceutical standards of manufacture – in many cases stricter than USA government requirements. Their Omnium Multivitamin/Mineral formula is excellent. Solgar products are available from top health-food stores, some chemists, and the Nutri Centre.

Beggars Lane
Aldbury

Tring
Herts HP23 5PT
UK
Tel: +44 (0) 1442 890 355
Fax: +44 (0) 1442 890 366
Website: **www.solgar.com**

Phyto Products Ltd

An excellent company for reasonably priced herbal tinctures and extracts. Originally set up to supply herbalists, every plant and herb they sell states the source of origin. Write to them for their price list.

Phyto Products Ltd

Park Works
Park House
Mansfield Woodhouse
Nottinghamshire NG19 8EF
UK
Tel: +44 (0) 1623 644 334
Fax: +44 (0) 1623 657 232

Specialist Herbal Supplies

This company has been supplying high-quality additive-free herbal aids to health practitioners in the UK and abroad since 1982. They now do a range of good-quality products for the general public as well, offering single herbs and mixtures as capsules, tinctures or extracts. Write to them for their catalogue.

Freepost (BR1396)
Brighton
East Sussex BN41 122
UK
Freephone (UK): 0800 542 5212
Fax: +44 (0) 1273 424 345
E-mail: **feedback@specialist-herbal.com**
Website: **www.herbalsupplies.com**

Bioforce (UK) Ltd

Suppliers of herbal extracts, tinctures, homeopathic remedies and natural self-care products and foods, Bioforce is a Swiss company started by the Swiss expert in natural health, Alfred Vogel. The company always use fresh herbs in preparing their products at the Bioforce factory in Roggwil. They do over 100 different herbal and homeopathic preparations, all of which are very high quality. They can be ordered by post but are often also available in good health-food stores and pharmacies carrying herbal products.

2 Brewster Place
Irvine
Ayrshire KA11 5DD
UK
Tel: +44 (0) 1294 277 344
Fax: +44 (0) 1294 277 922

Bio-Health Ltd

Bio-Health do an excellent range of single herbs, ointments and multi herb compounds in tablet and capsule form which you can purchase from good health food stores or order by post. Write to them for a catalogue.

Culpepper Close
Medway City Estate
Rochester
Kent ME2 4HU
UK
Tel: +44 (0) 1634 290 115
Fax: +44 (0) 1634 290 761
E-mail: **info@bio-health.co.uk**
Website: **www.bio-health.co.uk**

Herbal Apothecary

The Herbal Apothecary manufactures

and supplies the largest range of medicinal herbs in the UK, and for nearly 20 years has been the single largest supplier of herbal medicines to medical herbalists. They provide a wide range of plant and herbal products ranging from cut herbs to powders, tinctures, fluid extracts, creams, capsules and tablets together with essential oils.

103 High Street
Syston
Leicester LE7 1GQ
UK
Tel: +44 (0) 116 260 2690
Fax: +44 (0) 116 260 2757

Higher Nature Ltd

The Nutrition Centre
Burwash Common
East Sussex
TN19 7LX
Tel: +44 (0) 1435 884 668
Fax: +44 (0) 1435 883 720
E-mail: **info@higher-nature.co.uk**
Website: **www.higher-nature.co.uk**

BioCare

The Lakeside Centre
180 Lifford Lane
Kings Norton
Birmingham
West Midlands B30 3NT
UK
Tel: +44 (0) 121 433 3727
Fax: +44 (0) 121 433 3879
E-mail: **biocare@biocare.co.uk**
Website: **www.biocare.co.uk**

MSM Max

These MSM tablets are the purest and most potent form of MSM available – fast-acting and 100% pure with no additives or binders.

PO Box 33830
Portland
OR 97292
USA
Tel: +1 (503) 761 7450
Fax: +1 (503) 761 5383
Website: www.richdistributing.com

Also available from:
The Naturally Curious Company
P O Box 46
Pukekohe
Auckland 1800
New Zealand
Tel: +64 (9) 239 0496.
Fax: +64 (9) 239 0936
Website: www.naturalchoices.co.nz

Flaxseed Oil (Linseed oil)
Organic Flaxseed Oil is available from:

Savant Distribution Ltd
FREEPOST NEA 701
Leeds LS16 6YY
UK
Order line (UK): 08450 606070
Fax: +44 (0) 113 388 5248
E-mail: info@savant-health.com
Website: www.savant-health.com

Flower Essences
An excellent range of flower essences from all over the world is available from:

International Flower Essence Repertoire
The Living Tree
Milland
Nr Liphook
Hampshire GU30 7JS
UK
Tel: +44 (0) 1428 741 572
Fax: +44 (0) 1428 741 679

Bach Flower Remedies

Healing Herbs
PO Box 65
Hereford HR2 0UW
UK
Tel: +44 (0) 1873 890 218
Fax: +44 (0) 1873 890 314
These are Dr Edward Bach's range of flower remedies made to his original methodology.

Flower Essence Services (FES)
PO Box 1769
Nevada City
CA 95959
USA
Tel: +1 (530) 265 9136
Fax: +1 (530) 265 6467

Gabrielle Roth's Music
Available from good music stores, www.amazon.com and Gabrielle's own website www.ravenrecording.com

Omega-3s
Our favourite omega-3 oil supplement is made by Coromega. It comes in a sachet and is flavoured with orange. It's ideal for children. www.coromega.com.

Silica Gel
Our favourite is called Body Essential Silicea by H_bner. It is available from the Nutri Centre (see above).

RADIANCE EATING

Microfiltered Whey Protein
Solgar produce Whey To Go Protein Powder in vanilla, chocolate and mixed berry flavours. We especially like the chocolate and vanilla. BioPure Pure Protein by Metagenics or Twinlab's Super Whey Powder are also good. Our favourite, in terms of quality, not taste, is Medipro by Thorne Research. In addition to micro filtered whey, it contains a superbly balanced multivitamin and mineral complex – ideal as a meal-replacement smoothie. Whey To Go and BioPure can be purchased from the Nutri Centre.

Herb Teas
Some of our favourite blends include Cinnamon Rose, Orange Zinger and Emperors Choice by Celestial Seasonings: Warm & Spicy by Symmingtons and Creamy Carob French Vanilla. Yogi Tea by Golden Temple Products is a strong spicy blend, perfect as a coffee replacement. Green tea is available from health food stores and Oriental supermarkets.

Manuka Honey
Manuka honey should be easy to find in your local health food store. One of our favourites is 'Active' Manuka Honey from NatureBee as well as Comvita Manuka Honey, available from Xynergy Health Products.

Organics Direct
Offers a nationwide home delivery service of fresh vegetables and fruits, delicious breads, juices, sprouts, fresh soups, ready-made meals, snacks and baby foods. They also sell the state-of-the-art 2001 Champion Juicers and the 2002 Health Smart Juice Extractor for beginners. They even sell organic wines – all shipped to you within 24 hours.

Organics Direct
1-7 Willow Street

London EC2A 4BH
UK
Tel: +(44) 207 729 2828
Fax: +(44) 207 613 5800
Website: **www.organicsdirect.com**

Clearspring

Supply organic foods and natural remedies as well as macrobiotic foods by mail order. They have a good range of herbal teas, organic grains, whole seeds for sprouting, dried fruits, pulses, nut butters, soya and vegetable products, sea vegetables, drinks and Bioforce herb tinctures. Write to them for a catalogue:

Clearspring

Unit 19a, Acton Park Estate
London W3 7QE
UK
Tel: +44 (0) 208 749 1781
Fax: +(44) 208 746 2259
E-mail: **info@clearspring.co.uk**
Website: **www.clearspring.co.uk.**

Soya Milk

The best soya milk we have found is called Bonsoy. It is particularly good soya milk, unusual in that it is not packed in aluminium. It is organic and available from good health food stores. Try:

Fresh and Wild

196 Old Street
London EC1V 9FR
UK
Tel: +44 (0) 207 250 1708

Organic Meat

A UK Guide to where to buy organic meat

Organic Butchers

Crescent Consulting
1 The Crescent
Northampton, NN1 4SB
UK
Tel: +44 (0) 1604 459 962
Fax: +44 (0) 1604 459 963
www.organicbutchers.co.uk

Eastbrook Farms Organic Meat

This is our favourite supplier of all sorts of organic meat because they take such care over every order.

The Calf House

Cues Lane
Bishopstone
Swindon
Wiltshire, SN6 8PW
UK
Mail order: +44 (0) 1793 790 460.
Helpline: +44 (0) 1793 790 340
Fax: +44 (0) 1793 791 239
Email: **info@helenbrowningorganics.co.uk**
Website:
www.helenbrowningorganics.co.uk

Longwood Farm Organic Meats

Good-quality organic beef, pork, bacon, lamb, chicken, turkey, duck and geese, a variety of types of sausage, all dairy products, vegetables and organic groceries (2000 lines), are available mail order from:

Longwood Farm Organic Meats

Tuddenham St Mary,
Bury St Edmunds
Suffolk IP28 6TB
UK
Tel: +44 (0) 1638 717 120

Stevia

In most countries, not in the UK alas, stevia is readily available in health food stores in many forms. It comes as clear liquid extract in distilled water, powdered stevia leaf, as full strength (very sweet) stevioside extract. Our favourite kind, which we order from North America is called 'Stevita Spoonable Stevia.'

Water

We recommend the Fresh Water 1000 Water Filter System. It removes more than 90 percent of heavy metals, pesticides and hydrocarbons such as benzene, trihalmethanes, chlorine, oestrogen and bacteria without removing essential minerals like calcium. Available from:

The Fresh Water Filter Company Ltd

Gem House
895 High Road
Chadwell Heath
Essex, RM6 4HL
UK
Tel: +44 (0) 208 597 3223
Fax: +44 (0) 870 056 7264
E-mail: **mail@freshwaterfilter.com**
Website: **www.freshwaterfilter.com**

SKIN GLOW

The 'naturals'

These products are formulated primarily from natural ingredients. Most of them still contain parabens and other chemicals used as preservatives or for other purposes. However, these manufacturers are committed to producing cosmetics which are environmentally aware and as ecologically responsible as they can manage.

MSM Rich 'n Pure Lotion

Only natural ingredients are used in Dr. Rich's hydrating lotions. Designed specifically to help repair damage to your skin, they may be used by men and women alike. Your skin gradually develops a new softness and elasticity. This lotion contains 17 per cent Methyl Sulfonyl Methane (MSM) produced through distillation to ensure highest quality.
Website: **www.richdistributing.com**

Also available from:

The Naturally Curious Company, New Zealand

Tel: +64 (9) 239 0496
Fax +64 (9) 239 0936
Website: **www.naturalchoices.co.nz**

Scents of Balance

Kate Rossetto's unique American range of products includes a light-as-air Rose Silk Face Cream and 'Take Me There' emotional healing mists. These are high frequency sprays unique in their mood shifting and personal empowerment properties. Completely natural in formulation, they have also been infused with prayer and come in six varieties for different purposes: Forgiveness, Freedom, Power and Grace, Sweet Dreams, I Am, and Joy.

Kate Rossetto

Scents of Balance
2055 Andomeda Lane
Billings, MT 59105
USA
Tel: +1 (406) 2445 9182
E-mail: **kate@scentsofbalance.com**
Website: **www.scentsofbalance.com**

The Green People Company

Natural, certified organic skincare and toiletries.
Brighton Road
Handcross
West Sussex RH17 6BZ
UK
Mail order/enquiries: +44 (0) 1444 401 444
Fax: +44 (0) 1444 401 011
www.greenpeople.co.uk

AD®Skin/Synergy Nourishing Night Treatment

A wonderful nourishing gel which we like to use not only at night but as a base for mineral makeup application around the eyes.

AD®skin/synergy

P O Box 25595
London NW7 1WT
UK
Tel (UK): 0870 240 3350
E-mail: **amanda@amandadenningpr.co.uk**

Annemarie Börlind

C/O Simply Nature
Unit 7, Old Factory Buildings
Battenhurst Road
Stonegate
East Sussex TN5 7DU
UK
Tel: +44 (0) 1580 201687
Fax: +44 (00 1580 201697

Aubrey Organics (US)

4419 North Manhatten Avenue
Tampa FL 33614
USA
Tel: +1 (800) 282 7394
Fax: +1 (813) 876 8166
Website: **www.aubrey-organics.com**

Barefoot Botanicals

This is an excellent, small, range of highly ethical natural products.
Barefoot Botanicals Ltd.
282 St Paul's Road
London N1 2LH
UK
United Kingdom
Tel (UK): 0870 220 2273
Fax:+44 (00 1737 761632
E-mail: **salesuk@barefootbotanicals.com**
Website: **www.barefoot-botanicals.com**

Dr. Hauschka

Mail order (UK): +44 (0) 1386 792 622
Australia: +61 (2) 9666 2555
Can: +1 (440) 1386 792 622
E-mail: **enquiries@drhauschka.co.uk**
Website: **www.drhauschka.co.uk**
www.drhauschka.com

Weleda

Weleda grew out of the work of Rudolf Steiner and have been making medicines and body care products for 75 years. Weleda UK grow over 400 species of plants organically and biodynamically for use in their medicines and body care range. They do an excellent arnica cream and a delightful skincare range. Available from good health stores and pharmacies or order direct.

Weleda (UK) Ltd

Heanor Road
Ilkeston
Derbyshire DE7 8DR
UK
Tel: +44 (0) 115 944 8200
Fax +44 (0) 115 944 8210
Mail order/information: +44 (0) 115 9448 222
Websites: **www.weleda.co.uk**

www.weleda.com www.weleda.co.au
www.weleda.co.nz www.puritylife.com
(Canada)

Eve Lom's Cleanser

We both love Eve Lom's easy-to-use, oil based cleansing cream with essential oils. Just smooth it on then cleanse away dirt and make-up with the help of the mildly exfoliating muslin cloth that accompanies it. Available online from **www.evelom.co.uk**

The biological actives

This group of products contains nutraceuticals. They belong to the new wave of skincare which attempts to use vitamins and supplements like DMAE, alpha lipoic acid, Co Q10 and ALA to treat skin from the outside in. These products all contain chemical preservatives and conventionally formulated emulsions. Many of these are considered cosmeceuticals instead of cosmetics. In truth, there is no difference between the two. The name 'cosmeceuticals' is very often used to identify the kind of products you buy from a dermatologist or salon rather than what you buy over the counter in a store or pharmacy, but there is no legal definition of 'cosmeceuticals'.

Advanced Skin Therapy

This range has been formulated in the United States by Nuala Briggs. It is a large range, so you will need to pick and choose, depending on what your skin needs. They will ship anywhere.

Advanced Skin Therapy

42 Harley Street
London W1G 9PR

UK
Tel (UK): 07000 560 821

Also at
85 Main Road
Gidea Park
Essex RM2 5EL
UK
And
58 Weston Road
Brighton
East Sussex BN3 1JD
UK
E-mail: **hq@advancedskintherapy.co.uk**
Website: **www.advancedskintherapy.co.uk**

Environ

Leslie's favourite cosmetic range is Environ. Their products are specially formulated by South African plastic surgeon Dr Des Fernandes, a man who is without peer when it comes to using vitamins and neutraceuticals to transform skin. Fernandez has tremendous integrity reflected in everything he does and has won numerous awards both in surgery and for his range. Most of his Environ products are fragrance-free and all are free from colourants. All are highly effective – from the Proactive Rane based on Vitamin C and A to his top of the market Iozyme in which his new C-Quence Eye Gel and the other reformulated C-Quence products excel even his own previous creations. They are ideal for any woman wanting serious transformative, age-reversing skincare.

Head office

Environ® Skin Care
Access Park
Kenilworth

Cape Town
South Africa

PO Box 36057
Glosderry 7702
South Africa
Tel: +27 (21) 671 1467
Fax: +27 (21) 683 1016
E-mail: **factory@environ.co.za**

Distributed by:
Wholeview Ltd
Suite 29, Unit 1
1000 North Circular Road
London NW2 7JP
UK
Tel: +44 (0) 208 450 2020

Environ Skin Care Ltd.

62 Ladies Mile
Remuera
Auckland
New Zealand
Tel: +64 (9) 524 2005
Fax: +64 (9) 524 7042
E-mail: **environnz@xtra.co.nz**

Environ's Cosmetic Roll-Cit

Developed by Dr Des Fernandes, this is a revolutionary device in skincare treatments. The Roll-Cit is a roller riddled with minute needles which barely open the surface of the skin to allow deeper penetration of active ingredients. It is designed to help restore skin tightness, thicken the skin, soften facial lines, reduce scarring, and to speed up the disappearance of pigmentation marks.

Art A Face

A favourite of plastic surgeons, this range is based on colostrum which has wonderful healing properties after surgery or peels. Their fragrance is

Acknowledgements

We are grateful to all of the authentic women and men who have helped us bring this book to birth: to David Eldridge for his inspiration and his endless devotion to the task of creating its design and getting the visuals right. To Yvette Brown – The Fox – for her indefatigable commitment to its editing and her going far beyond the call of duty. To Carey Smith for her willingness to take on a project mid-stream, her flexibility and her enthusiasm. To Natalie Hunt for her endless care and efficiency. And finally to our friends – these authentic woman who contributed to the book by allowing us to photograph them just as they are – perfect, every one: Suzanna Erickson, Stephanie Gardiner, Regan Hyde, Lada Kenton-Dau, Eva Mason, and Leneke Pearson. For us it has been a great pleasure to know and work with each one of you. Thank you.

Leslie and Susannah

About the Authors

LESLIE KENTON

Award-winning writer, photographer, television broadcaster and teacher Leslie Kenton is well known throughout the English-speaking world for her no-nonsense approach and is highly respected for her in-depth reporting. Her fans are legion. 'One expert who can genuinely be described as both pioneering and visionary', Leslie has been a consultant to the European Parliament for the Green Party and a course developer for Britain's Open University. She has written more than three dozen bestselling books on health, beauty and spirituality, delivered the McCarrison Lecture at the Royal Society of Medicine, received the PPA Technical Writer of the Year award, and conceived and created the worldwide Origins skincare range for cosmetic giant Estée Lauder. Leslie Kenton insists that authentic power and freedom come from *within* and the only true 'guru' is the individual human soul.

SUSANNAH KENTON

Susannah's writing career began at age 18 when she co-authored the bestselling *Raw Energy*. The book's success led to her starring in a TV cookery series, hosting a weekly health/beauty TV spot, and writing several more books including the teenage handbook *Dare to be You*. After graduating from Columbia University in New York, Susannah studied acting in London. She then pursued her passion for theatre in Paris where she worked for seven years as an actress and singer. In 1996 she moved to Los Angeles. While continuing her work in the performing arts, Susannah also immersed herself in the healing arts, becoming qualified as a nutritional consultant, teaching workshops on creativity and facilitating sacred circles. Through her writing, workshops and performance, Susannah is dedicated to exploring and celebrating the full potential of the authentic self.